your whole life

The 3D Plan for
• Eating Right
• Living Well
• Loving God

Carol Showalter
with Maggie Davis
MS, RD, LDN, FADA, CDE

Devotionals revised and edited
by Martin Shannon

PARACLETE PRESS
BREWSTER, MASSACHUSETTS
3D

Your Whole Life is the new 3D plan for
eating right, living well, and loving God.
3D (Diet, Discipline and Discipleship),
a Christ-centered health program founded in
1972 by Carol Showalter, has helped
over one million people.

Dear Reader,

This book is not intended to replace the expert advice that may be needed for your unique health issues. If you have specific medical nutritional needs, such as diabetes, a severe cardiac condition, a metabolic disorder, gastrointestinal disease, an eating disorder, or any other serious medical condition, it's important for you to seek the advice of your own Registered Dietitian, Licensed Nutritionist, Certified Diabetes Educator, Physician, or another qualified healthcare professional before making significant changes to either your diet or your exercise regime.

Carol Showalter

Contents

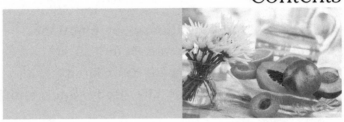

Part Three A New Creation

For additional resources go to
www.3DYourWholeLife.com

- Recommended Daily Portion Guidelines
- Weight and Target Food Intake Level
- Your Weight History Questionnaire
- Waist and Hips Measurement
- Food Record
- Menu Ideas and Recipes
- Testimonials
- 3D Groups Directory
- Monthly newsletterre
- Information

Introduction

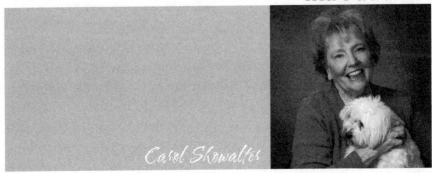

Carol Showalter

THIRTY-FIVE YEARS AGO the first Christian diet program began, and soon it swept across the United States and many other countries. As the director of 3D, I wrote a book about the program, with sales reaching more than 500,000 copies.

The 3D program came out of my own personal need. I was a young minister's wife, with four children and many church responsibilities. I found that I could not cope with all the demands on my life. So I called out to God to help me. He heard my cry, and 3D was launched. This program was touched by the hand of God, and it continues to change lives wherever and whenever someone picks up a copy of the book or the devotions. That is because 3D is more than a diet program. It is a program about living a whole life. And I have found wholeness as, to the best of my ability, I have lived the principles that were set forth in that book.

When I realized last November that we would be bringing out a new book, I knew God would hold me accountable. For years I have been a walker and a swimmer, but I knew that I needed even more exercise. So I bought a treadmill, and I began taking exercise more seriously. I also bought a pedometer and began counting exactly how many steps I was taking in a day. I renewed my prayer for the people in the 3D program around the world and thanked God for holding this program in his hands all these years. And I began to ask God just exactly what this new book should be.

Although I have changed over the past 35 years, I am as passionate today as I was in the beginning of 3D about the vision of what can happen when people earnestly consider the whole person and not just the body. I am as convinced as ever that committed Christians are being challenged to look at the connection between the body and the soul. We must join with each other. Our health, our emotions, and our energy are all involved with our Christian walk. How can we do this better? We believe that in this book we have some answers that will move us along this journey.

> I am as passionate today as I was in the beginning of 3D about the vision of what can happen when people earnestly consider the whole person and not just the body.

As *Your Whole Life* is launched, I am filled with the burning excitement I had in the beginning, because I expect God to work in my life just as he will in yours. Though I am older now, I have the same need to want more of God and less of me. I am not interested in dieting, I am interested in eating right.

The 3Ds are Diet, Discipline, and Discipleship. I would like to define these terms with a new understanding: Eating Right (Diet), Living Well (Discipline), and Loving God (Discipleship). I challenge you to turn your head and your heart around to a new direction with one goal: to become *whole*.

Every year in the late fall I receive phone calls from writers and editors of the most popular women's magazines. This is what they often say: "We are doing a feature on faith-based diet programs and wonder if you can give me the names and phone numbers of women around the country that have lost at least half their body weight in 3D. And also we will need photos of before and after."

The first few years we worked hard to find names and numbers and make contacts so that 3D could have publicity in national women's magazines. Then I began to realize that these magazines wanted something else as well: they wanted only pretty faces, and wanted only those of a certain age bracket. They didn't tell me that on the phone, but after a while I began to ask them directly if that criteria was essential. With great hesitation they would tell me that those qualities very definitely would be important. (Take a look at the magazines at the grocery checkout counter this week. You'll see what I mean.)

Last year I finally told one of those magazine editors that although I would like to comply with her request, it really went against everything that 3D has stood for. I stymied her because I didn't want to give her the names of the 3D "success" crowd. I have always been candid with every reporter and have told my age, and have made it clear that I am still fighting the weight battle. I never received anything but respect for my honesty. But now it was time for me to stand up for the integrity of 3D.

> Although I would like to comply with her request, it really went against everything that 3D has stood for.

That editor wrote me several e-mails saying how sorry she was that she couldn't use 3D program members, because she had read my book and loved what I was saying—so, she asked, would I please reconsider. "Your program does not center on being thin, and that's the story I want to tell—but also with pictures of your successes." I could not say yes, because to do so would have compromised my convictions. And we finished our e-mail correspondence with mutual respect for each other.

These experiences with magazines in recent years have prompted me to create this new 3D book and program, *Your Whole Life.*

In my walk toward good health I have benefited tremendously over the past six years from the wisdom of well-known nutritionist and registered dietitian Maggie Davis. I went to Maggie for help with diet, but I got more than nutritional help. Maggie put many questions before

> I went to Maggie for help with diet, but I got more than nutritional help.

me that pushed me to examine my whole life—questions that to her were obviously related to my weight struggle. So I did some spiritual inventory at the same time that I was learning new facts about nutrition. Maggie agreed to join me in this new book and share with readers her wisdom about eating right, living well, and loving God, and how these things indeed work together.

This new edition is chock full of new concepts and a new understanding about nutrition and "diet." It is about transformation from the inside out, and it is about feeling good about yourself from the outside in! It has challenges for each one of us about what it means to live well and how to incorporate these changes into our daily lives.

THE BOOK THAT YOU ARE HOLDING IN YOUR HANDS today is one of reflection, understanding, and new challenges. It will challenge you to face yourself just the way you are. It will challenge you to come anew to a place where you can accept yourself, weaknesses and all, and to know beyond a shadow of doubt that God can help you. It will also challenge you to believe in the love and forgiveness of God, who is in the business of making all things new. There is no time to waste in looking back and counting our failures and wishing that we could have done things differently. That is all in God's hands. Now it is time to stand in the present and to look forward with open minds and hearts to new insights and new beginnings. Remember, God promises that the best is yet to come.

Many new insights and challenges will come from Maggie, who is walking alongside to share what she has taught me and so many others. *Your Whole Life* is our response to the millions of people who have gone through the 3D program or other diet programs, and still have questions and want to learn more about living well and becoming whole. Maggie brings forward new concepts and offers them through the interpretive framework of the 3D plan; her nutritional and wellness advice are presented in shaded sections of the book.

You will also encounter spiritual readings, devotions, hymns, and other forms of encouragement that have been tested through the ages by men and women of God. There are "Tips for Men" that speak specifically to men's concerns in the area of wellness and nutrition. And there are guidelines for anyone reading this book who would like to start a group.

This book is divided into a twelve-week program with a different challenge for each week. Take your time reading *Your Whole Life*.

You can follow the 3D plan by yourself, or others can join you and form a support group where you can help each other, as we did in the first days of 3D. Guidelines for group leaders can be found on pages 278–279 of this book, and also on our website, www.3DYourWholeLife. com. As you move through the pages of this book, it is my prayer that you will see the concepts, challenges, and knowledge as tools for your own success. But don't expect anything in here to be *the* answer. Make a twelve-week commitment right now to this program. Be open to new understandings of your weight struggles; be honest about your needs; and most of all, have *faith*.

> Jesus says to a woman, "Your faith has made you whole."

God is in the business of healing lives, and you are at the top of his list today. The Scripture verse that led us to the title of this book was one in which Jesus says to a woman, "Your faith has made you whole" (Mark 5:34, cs). We believe this, and we hope you will, too.

Carol Showalter

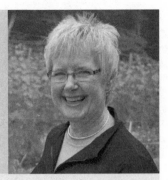

Maggie Davis

WHEN I FIRST BEGAN MY PRIVATE PRACTICE AS A NUTRITIONIST, I was often discouraged when working with people who needed to lose weight. I was trained to give people diets, including menus, recipes, and the like. I was educated to tell them what to eat, but within a few years I realized that this sort of approach simply didn't work. Attempting to follow restrictive "one-size-fits-all" menus often leads to repeated cycles of quick loss, then regaining all or more of the weight, followed by outright despair at the process.

Scientific evidence continues to document the dismal, long-term results of most weight loss programs. Repeated rounds of "dieting" erode the health of those who seek to become as slim as models we see in the media, trying and failing many times in their lives. Each new diet plan promises that if you refrain from eating a particular set of foods, you will be successful. Just the opposite seems to be true: you need balance. My objective is to help you find a way to include all types of whole and healthy foods, as well as occasional treats or splurges, while attaining or maintaining a healthy body weight. My goal is to educate you and inspire you to eat right for your whole life.

Long ago, I abandoned the use of rigid diets with my clients and adopted a system for gradual changes that are positive, practical, and likely to become permanent.

Long ago, I abandoned the use of rigid diets with my clients and adopted a system for gradual changes that are positive, practical, and likely to become permanent. I don't usually know at the outset of treatment exactly what will work for a client, or how long the treatment will be needed. The first step is to get to know what and how a person eats. You will be doing this for yourself. It is also important to explore the why's of eating. In what sort of situations do you eat right, or not eat right?

The remaining work is a process that involves incorporating small but significant changes, applying food and nutrition knowledge, dealing with the obstacles and challenges, and continued self-knowledge. Over the years I have seen that those who are successful in eating right and managing their weight for many years are the ones who bring mind, body, and spirit into their work.

And work it is! The work can take anywhere from several months or years to a lifetime, being aware that treatment and intervention may be necessary again at various points in the future. I might add that my patients and clients have included individuals from nearly every ethnic and religious background. They have included people of faith as well as people who do not practice religion, but one thing they have in common is that they have experienced spiritual battles that involved food. They have collectively taught me that it takes a whole person to make a whole life.

So it is very exciting to be involved in a program that incorporates the whole person into the process. It is as if Carol Showalter and I have been working in parallel for the past 35 years: I, as a nutrition professional in a community setting, and Carol, as a dieter in her own life and as a spiritual teacher through her books and through thousands of 3D groups across the world. We have had similar discoveries that we want to share with you.

Nutritional Starting Points

Food and nutrition are the **foundation of good health,** and *Your Whole Life* provides a nutritional program with the tools you need to eat right for your whole life. The "Eating Right" part of this program is based on the Dietary Guidelines for Americans, food pyramid recommendations, as well as on my work with individuals and weight loss groups. It is intended for use by women and men eighteen years of age or older. (Younger teens should consult a nutritional professional before making any significant changes to their diet.)

Although the dietary guidelines and food pyramid recommend specific ranges of various types of food, there are many ways of successfully applying such guidelines. *Your Whole Life* also incorporates a method of **self-assessment and gradual behavior change** that I have used in my practice with individuals and groups for nearly 35 years. We will work together so that you learn to develop personal goals and strategies for improving your food habits, implement changes, identify barriers to eating right, and ultimately establish a system for making healthy food choices to last a lifetime.

During this process, you will learn not only to enjoy eating right but also how to know yourself in a deeper and more meaningful way. This is a journey as much is it is a destination. There will be **speed bumps, stop signs**, and detours on the road— but you will use this program to keep you traveling on your journey to eating right and achieving better health.

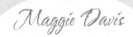

give yourself PERMISSION

If you have children, or if remember your own experiences as a child, the concept of the permission slip will be very familiar to you. Maybe you have signed many of these in the past.

Some of us—most often women—need to give ourselves permission to take care of our bodies, minds, and spirits. Often, we consume our time and energies with caring for others, and we neglect ourselves. We even convince ourselves that this is good—we might even tell ourselves that we are being better Christians by disregarding our own needs. But you need to know that this is *not* good. God wants you to care for this body that he called a "temple of the Holy Spirit within you" (1 Corinthians 6:19), and he wants you to be his child. Pause for a moment, and actually give yourself permission to spend these next twelve weeks caring for yourself.

What Are the 3Ds?

diet EATING RIGHT

The word *diet* does not actually mean losing weight. Diet means eating habits—*what* you eat. What do *you* eat every day? What is your diet? Think about this word in a new way as you delve into the 3D plan for the next twelve weeks. By the end of this program you will have a new understanding of the word *diet*. And it won't be such a negative force in your life.

You have probably picked up this book—and wanted this information—because you want to lose weight. And the word that drew your attention to the book was *diet*. For this reason, the first of the three D's has always referred to eating and changing our habits of eating. But this is not at all a typical diet book. I promise you that you will learn how to eat right, and if you faithfully incorporate these principles into your life over the next twelve weeks, you will certainly lose weight, but you will also come to understand your life in a whole new way.

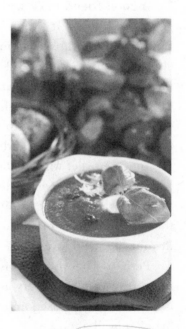

The word *diet* does not actually mean losing weight.

You don't "go on a diet" in the 3D plan. Instead, you work with God to bring your life under his will and guidance. This does not mean that God wants you to be skinny; and it

> You don't "go on a diet" in the 3D plan.

doesn't mean that if you were more godly you would be skinny. God wants you to be whole. But it is important that you face the fact that the struggle is between accepting yourself as overweight, or being willing to battle all of the factors involved in making hard choices.

A good friend once said to me: "You can go to bed fat, or you can go to bed hungry. It's your choice." I found that a shocking statement! But it is one of those statements that I think about often. Many of my choices happen at the end of a long day. Will I stick the tablespoon into the half-gallon ice cream container in the freezer, will I grab a few candies from the candy dish in the living room, will I pop a chocolate chip cookie into my mouth on the way through the kitchen? Or will I resist these temptations and feel like I am going to bed hungry?

Your new diet will be about developing eating habits that will help you lose weight. Expect to lose weight. It *will* happen. But don't forget the important issue of finding your true self and knowing more about the love of God no matter what you weigh. That issue has to be settled in your life. God loves you!

Perhaps what you need is not so much another diet as guidance and support in ordering every aspect of your life as a child of God. If that is how you feel, please join us for twelve weeks, because that is what the 3D plan is all about!

THOUGHT ❝ God be in my head, and in my understanding.

God be in my eyes, and in my looking.

God be in my mouth, and in my speaking.

God be in my heart and in my thinking.

God be at my end, and at my departing. ❞

(Old Sarum Primer, 1558, Salisbury, England)

A New Diet

n our culture, diet has more commonly come to have the meaning of a special, restrictive, or therapeutic regimen of eating to treat excess weight gain or a particular medical condition. But these sorts of diets are usually temporary. People go "on" and "off" popular diets; they never last forever. **When Carol and I use the word** *diet,* **we are referring to your daily way of eating.**

We all consume a diet that is unique to ourselves. In my practice, I have never seen two individuals, even twins, who eat exactly the same foods, in the same amounts, day in and day out. Your diet is made up of the foods you eat on a typical day, most days of your life. It consists of the type and amount of food you eat, the food you cook at home (and the food that you taste while making dinner), the food you order for take-out, the snacks you eat at work or in the car. Your journal and action plan will consider all of these factors.

As part of the 3D plan of eating right, you first need to evaluate where, when, why, and how you are eating now. What is your diet like today? You also need to assess your health and your fitness level. You will want to examine your previous attempts to change your eating habits and determine what you have learned. **What helped you in the past? What didn't? What led you to abandon your previous attempts?** These are important questions that can help you to gain insight before attempting changes now. Just as professional athletes examine videotapes of their past performances, you will benefit from looking back at your eating behaviors and seeing where you could do better in the future. Since no experience in life is ever wasted, what you considered failed attempts at dieting in the past may hold the key to your progress in the future.

This program will include setting realistic long- and short-term goals for your health and weight. You need goals that are positive, practical, and permanent. Unlike diets that promise that you will "Lose 10 pounds in 10 days," you will be developing realistic goals for yourself and no one else.

You will be developing goals for this particular phase of your life, knowing that in the future you will probably need to review and revise them. Sometimes I liken eating right to making a good financial investment for your future or your retirement. What you eat can affect your life now and in the future with dividends of good health, but the deposits need to be made gradually, with sound advice and regular re-evaluation of your goals. In short, eating right each day can be an important contribution to your nutritional IRA.

Maggie Davis

discipline LIVING WELL

Hebrews 12:11 says that no *discipline* is pleasant at the time, but rather is painful. But the verse also promises that discipline will produce righteousness. So it connects the idea of discipline—which some of us see only as negative—with what is positive: the promise of a righteous life. Discipline is the second key to wholeness; it is part of an integrated life.

I recently returned from a pilgrimage. I call my trip a pilgrimage for two reasons: first, because I visited many religious sites in Germany and Italy; and second, because I did some of it by myself. I walked through towns and cities and into churches, and my pedometer was counting, counting, counting, and my steps were many. But I also felt that I was on a deeply spiritual journey on the inside. My pedometer could not record the steps I was taking spiritually, but those inward steps were just as real as the outward ones.

Throughout the trip, somewhere in my heart, I knew that I was definitely learning discipline. It may not seem that traveling to beautiful places is a form of discipline, but for me, it was. In those unique settings, I was practicing living well. I was feeding my body beautiful, local foods; I was exercising my body with many steps of walking; my eyes were observing so much beauty; and my heart was responding to the overwhelming mystery of God in places like the catacombs of Rome.

Most of all, as I walked, prayed, and visited sites, I found myself in continual conversations with God. I would say, "Thank you for this gift of such a trip," and I would ask, "What do I need to know about you in all of this, God?" "What should I visit next?" "Should I walk, should I take a taxi, should I eat now or later?" My dialogue with God was unceasing.

Then I returned home. And even though the marvelous trip to Germany and Italy had ended, deep inside my heart, I know that this very journey was exactly what God plans for me daily—regardless of where I am. He wants me to enjoy beautiful food; he wants me to see the trees and the flowers and the water all around me—these aspects of nature that awe me and show me the mystery of God; he wants me to turn to him for every direction I take; he wants me to care for my body through exercise. In short, he wants me to *live well*. To live this way is possible—but it takes discipline.

> Deep inside my heart, I know that this very journey was exactly what God plans for me daily—regardless of where I am.

discipleship LOVING GOD

Webster's dictionary defines *disciple* as one who follows his or her master. Throughout this book, you will find pointers to assist you toward discipleship; and discipleship points you toward God, your true master. God is the most necessary component of a whole life—and that is what the average diet plan misses.

A soldier goes to boot camp and undergoes the rigors of training to succeed as a soldier. The athlete trains to attain a prize. The farmer rises early and labors long and hard to obtain a good harvest. Whatever we practice long enough becomes a part of us. So let's practice the wisdom of God. The words and the life of faith will become a part of you on this journey of twelve weeks.

Right now, we encourage you to enter into an important spiritual practice. Make a commitment to stick with the thoughts and the plans of this program for twelve weeks. That's a spiritual commitment, and this is where *Your Whole Life* differs from other "diet" books. The spiritual insight and emphasis are the most important parts of this book and program, and they are essential to your success.

Commit to keep these regular practices over the course of the next twelve weeks:

■ **Read the devotions for each day.** Included in this book are seven days' worth of devotions for each week. Resist the temptation to read ahead—something we tend to do when delving into a new program. Take this process slowly to ensure that the spiritual lessons can take root in your life. Every day we want you to have encouragement from the wisdom of God, as expressed in Scripture and in the thoughts of others.

■ **Memorize Scripture.** As adults, we sometimes turn away from this sort of activity. You may even still remember verses you memorized as a child, but just as you put away your bicycle, you may have stopped memorizing God's Word. As you learn the Scripture verses, you will realize the profound effect they will have on all aspects of your life. Find ways to make this memorizing fun—as if you were learning a new recipe. Maybe you can even memorize Scripture together with others!

■ **Pray for five people by name each morning.** These can be family members or co-workers. If you are in a 3D group, be sure to include those friends.

■ **Write in your journal** the insights you are gaining in your whole life each day.

THOUGHT 66 God always heals us,
and with the most amazing gentleness over time.
It does take time for us to heal in ways
that will bring God the most glory,
and us the most joy, forever. 99

(Julian of Norwich, 1342-ca. 1416)

How 3D Began

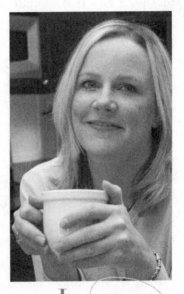

WEIGHT USED TO OBSESS ME. Whether I was gaining or losing, I was thinking about my weight most of the time. In fact, that was the first thing I noticed about other people, so I was convinced that weight was the first thing they noticed about me. And I'd judged overweight people for years. I was quite proud that I could lose weight successfully. But I never stopped to face the cold fact that I gained weight just as successfully every year.

I was very upset one night as I walked into the room for a Weight Watchers meeting. I had been there before. There were fat women all over the place. Some were sitting down, gabbing away; others were waiting in lines for one thing or another. Three women in the room, out of fifty or sixty, had thinner figures. And two of these were sitting at the table, registering people for class.

I walked into the room for a Weight Watchers meeting. I had been there before.

The class was being held in my church in Rochester, New York. Parkminster Presbyterian Church was one of Rochester's rapidly growing young congregations, and my husband, Bill, was the senior minister. We lived directly across the street from the church. For several minutes I had been watching fat ladies get out of cars and walk into the East Hall before getting up the courage to walk over myself. I took my place in the line of women waiting to register.

The weight battle had been going on in my life for a long time—over ten years. In the course of a year I would gain twenty or twenty-five pounds, and then in two or three months I would lose them any way I could. I had tried all kinds of crash diet programs that sometimes worked and sometimes didn't. I would eat only one thing for three or four weeks and usually lose the weight pretty quickly. (One time I ate only beets for three weeks!)

> I had tried all kinds of crash diet programs.

Two years earlier, I had gone to see my doctor for my yearly checkup. "Mrs. Showalter?" I put my magazine down and stood up to follow a nurse with a clipboard in her hand. "Would you come this way, please?" I followed closely behind her, trying to be amiable, but she was all business. "Beautiful day, isn't it?" I suggested. No response.

She stopped abruptly at the gray monster—the hospital scale outside the doctor's office. "Please step up here, so I can check your weight for the doctor." I started to take off my shoes, but she said, "That isn't necessary, Mrs. Showalter, it won't make much difference." Well, I knew she was wrong! Shoes *do* make a difference, and so does the time of day and several other things, but there was no sense in arguing with her. I'd just deduct in my own mind what I thought those shoes weighed and also a pound or so because it was the middle of the afternoon, and I always weighed more at that time.

The bottom weight indicator was set in the 100-pound (45-kilo) notch. She pushed the top weight to the far right. Nothing happened; the balance bar at the end of the scale cleaved to the top—147, 148, 150, still nothing. "Looks like we'll have to move up a notch," she remarked casually. That meant into the 150-pound (68-kilo) notch. If only she had let me take off my shoes.

The clunk of the weight as she changed it seemed to echo all over the waiting room. I was sure everyone heard it for a mile around. She kept moving the top weight, but still nothing happened. My eyes were glued to the balance bar; when would it detach itself from the top? Oh, no, 160, 165, and now finally a slight movement, and slowly it began to descend. I was 167 pounds (76 kilos) and devastated. I expected that I would be over 150 pounds (68 kilos), but never did I dream I was back up there—again.

My doctor was angry when he read the chart. "Get that weight off, Carol, and quickly! You're too young to weigh almost 170 pounds." I didn't say anything, but inside I was furious. Who did he think he was? I was there for my gynecological checkup, not a lecture on weight control. "As soon as you leave here today, I want you to find the diet group nearest to your house and join it right away. Like Weight Watchers or Diet Workshop. Either of those near you?"

I dearly wished I could have lied at that point. But I paused and gulped noticeably. "Yes, Weight Watchers has two groups that meet in our church every week." "Well, there can't be anything more convenient," he said with a smile. But he wouldn't just drop it. He went on to talk about how young mothers fall into depression from being overweight, and how older people can die from being overweight, and on and on.

I was insulted and angry, but his confrontation worked. The next week was when I joined Weight Watchers—the first time. To my chagrin I weighed in at 167 pounds (76 kilos) that first meeting—without my shoes and before breakfast! And the program worked for me. The first twenty pounds went quickly, and then I got comfortable and lazy for a while. I thought I looked pretty good at 147 pounds (67 kilos), and I was not as anxious to get the rest off. In fact it wasn't until fifteen months after I joined that I graduated at 130 pounds (59 kilos). Naturally, I was totally convinced that I would never, never gain weight again. Finally, I knew how and what to eat. It would be easy from here on—or so I thought.

But here I was again, standing in line at Weight Watchers, waiting to register once more. The line had been moving steadily, and soon I was facing the thin registration clerk. She told me to fill out the front and back questions on the payment book and said the weekly fee was $2.50, in addition to a five-dollar registration fee. "Does it make any difference that I'm a graduate of this program?" I asked quietly. (I never would have mentioned it, but I had a hunch the cost was less for ex-members.) "Oh," she said, looking up at me, perhaps trying to remember my face. "Do you have your lifetime membership book with you?" "No, I'm sorry, and I haven't the vaguest idea what I did with it. I hadn't planned on using it again," I mumbled.

I hated the humiliation of needing Weight Watchers, and its membership certificate was not something I treasured. I had buried it somewhere and quickly forgotten about it. "I'll look in our files and see if we have your old registration number and weight chart, Mrs. Showalter. In the meantime, why don't you just step over to the other line and wait to be weighed in."

The weigh-in line was moving towards one of the room dividers. There were voices behind the divider, but the conversations were not discernible. "Next, please," were the only words that clearly came over the top of the partition. While I was still standing there, the clerk brought me my new book. "You don't have to pay the registration fee, Mrs. Showalter," she said, handing me back a five-dollar bill. "And if, I mean, when, you get within two pounds of your goal, you will no longer have to pay the weekly fee, either. Those are the privileges of our graduates," she said, smiling and giving a plug for the program to those within earshot.

Soon the "Next, please" was for me. I stepped behind the divider and handed my book to a slender, gray-haired woman. She didn't even bother to look up. I was only a number to her. "Step on the scale, please." "Can't I take off my shoes?" I pleaded. "Of course," she answered.

Weighing-in over, I chose a seat on the end of the very last row, trying not to be seen. I began to look around the room for objects of interest. Bible verses were written on blackboards, and Sunday school papers were tacked up on the various partitions. One partition caught my attention: a big, red smiley face was painted right on the rough finish of the partition. The face was trimmed widely with black paint, and beside it there were large, bold words: Smile, God Has The Answer. I couldn't take my eyes off those words. Smile—I wasn't in the mood. "If God has the answer, why am I here?" I asked myself.

That smile sign was disgustingly persistent. It made me angry. I knew God has answers for lots of problems, but he had never helped me with my weight problem! Yes, answers for searching teenagers, answers for troubled marriages, answers for big problems, but. . . .

> Smile, God Has The Answer. I couldn't take my eyes off those words. Smile— I wasn't in the mood.

I squirmed. "Hey, preacher's wife, won't your God help you? Can't you practice what you preach to so many others?" The thoughts coming at me from the potent sign were like poison darts.

But I *had* prayed. Many, many nights I had prayed. Falling asleep, I would beg God to please take away my desire for the fattening S's— sweets, snacks, and seconds! But I would wake up and hardly be able to wait until breakfast to take the first bite of a doughnut. Then after breakfast, I'd remember God and throw up a quick prayer, asking him to keep all temptations away from me throughout the day, quickly quoting the verse in 1 Corinthians that said, "There has no temptation overtaken you but such as is common to man. But God is faithful and just and will not allow you to be tempted above that which you are able to bear. . . ." Now it was up to God to just keep those temptations away from me. The responsibility was on him. But everywhere I turned, I would bump smack into moist chocolate chip cookies, sticky sweet rolls, and filled candy dishes.

The speaker was an attractive woman of about thirty-five. I had seen her buzzing around the room and assumed that she was the lecturer. She had the best figure in the room, and the way she was dressed and the way she strutted around, it was obvious that it was a relatively new figure of which she was proud. I was jealous of it.

"Before we get too far into today's meeting," she went on, "I have something for you to see: a picture of me three summers ago." She flashed an enlarged picture of herself draped over a chaise lounge eating a piece of cake and drinking something out of a can. The fat was hanging off her lifted arm, and she was bulging over the sides of the chaise lounge. It was hard to believe that it was really her. "I've lost 106 pounds [48 kilos] and have kept just about all of it off for almost three years now. And if I can do it, so can you!"

For the next ten minutes, she talked about the emotional and medical dangers for fat people, emphasizing her points with a handmade flip chart filled with statistics. I was bored, and I tuned her out. That smiley face was still grinning at me, and I was pouting back at it.

Suddenly the thought struck me: was God trying to say something to me through that sign? Perhaps half an hour had passed since I first had seen that big red face and those five words. Maybe God had an answer for me I hadn't heard before. I had no idea what it could be.

The lecturer continued. Names were being called now, with an announcement of how much weight each person had lost that week. There was laughter and clapping after each name, but I was not a part of it. I was busy making a decision. "All new members must stay after the class for a few minutes, so that I can explain some of the details of the diet," she said, pointing to the side of the room I was sitting on. "We'll meet over there. The rest of you are free to go now. Have a good week, everyone," she said, waving goodbye.

While the majority of the women headed towards the door, six or seven were making their way to the rows she had pointed to. I got up and headed for the door myself. I could almost feel the lecturer's eyes on my back. At that moment I had no idea what I was going to do about my weight problem after I walked out that door. But I knew God was going to help me—somehow. He *did* have the answer. And as I slipped out the door, just before it closed, I was almost smiling.

I felt peaceful by the time I reached home. And I began to see some things about myself: I had to stop putting the blame on God for not answering my prayers. The problem was me, not God. I loved to eat—I just hated to gain weight. And even after "willing" the weight off through Weight Watchers, I still chose to begin eating the wrong foods again. And no amount of praying in the morning or at night was going to magically wash those Calories away. If I ate what I wanted, when I wanted to, I was going to get fat again. It was as simple as that. The problem was not God, nor was it with the Weight Watchers program. The problem was me! And it was about time I faced that.

isn't a good christian SUPPOSED TO DO EVERYTHING RIGHT?

In the months that followed that October morning in 1972, I found that my weight problem no longer consumed my thoughts, yet at the same time I didn't try to avoid it. I was still heavier than I should have been, but I was peaceful. And there was something else: My compulsive eating seemed to stop. I wasn't losing, but I wasn't gaining, either.

Almost before I knew it, fall and winter had passed, and spring was upon us. The women of the church began to plan their annual spring luncheon. The date was May 3, and women from all over the community were invited. The guest speakers were two women who were not strangers to our congregation, Mrs. Cay Andersen and Mrs. Judy Sorensen.

Bill and I had first heard Cay and Judy, as they were popularly known, twelve years earlier at a Faith at Work conference in Massachusetts. They had shared how God had called them, in a little church on Cape Cod, to minister together as a team, counseling and leading retreats at various churches around New England. Cay's husband, Bill, was a builder, and they owned and operated a beautiful guesthouse at Rock Harbor, near Orleans, with their son, Peter. They led a relatively peaceful life. Although Cay had been very sick for several years, she was now able to manage the guesthouse. The Sorensen family, Judy and her husband, also named Bill, and their four children vacationed on Cape Cod every year. Before long, the Sorensens moved in with the Andersens at Rock Harbor—four adults and five children under one roof. The teaching that Cay and Judy did was based largely on the experiences they were having in living out the Christian life under these circumstances.

Our first reaction to their sharing was mixed. My husband was unimpressed with their lack of formal Christian training, and yet they intrigued him. "They're so spontaneous!" I exclaimed. "They don't seem to prepare their talks, and they don't seem to know who is going to speak first or say what." We came away not quite knowing what to make of these two ladies from Cape Cod.

The luncheon came off as an unqualified success, as Cay and Judy shared from their lives. The 250 guests were moved alternately to laughter and to solemn reflection. That luncheon marked only the beginning of a wonderful week of learning and growth for a great many people at Parkminster Church, including me.

I'm a judgmental person. I didn't like it, for example, when the women serving the luncheon that day failed to serve the head table first. And I didn't like the serving dishes they had picked to use. I wanted to look good in front of Cay and Judy, and I wanted the church to look good, so those things and more irritated me. But as Cay and Judy began to talk about judgments and how destructive they were, I listened. And before long, tears were rolling down my cheeks through the rest of their talk. It was as if they had been aware of my thoughts during lunch. The more they talked, the more distressed I became. It wasn't just the thoughts I had at this luncheon that troubled me—I now saw that I was judging others all the time.

I could not stop crying. Even when everyone else was laughing, I could hardly get a full smile on my face. I wasn't sure I was going to be able to make it through the luncheon. And I was embarrassed. I tried brushing my tears away as inconspicuously as possible—praying no one would notice. After all, I was the senior minister's wife, and I had to keep my poise in front of 250 women! Or so I thought. Bill was arranging private counseling sessions after the luncheon, for those who wanted to talk with Cay and Judy. "Do you think I could see them first?" I whispered to him. I felt that I had to divulge my judgments to Cay and Judy quickly, before I could be of any use to Bill or the church or my family. So I became the first in line for private counseling in the chapel.

The moment I walked in and saw them, I burst out crying. "I'm a mess and I really need help!" "Here, Carol," Judy said, smiling and handing me a Kleenex. "What seems to be going on in you?"

THOUGHT   66 If we had no faults of our own,
we would take much less pleasure
in complaining about those of others. 99
François Fénelon, 1651–1715

I expected a two-hour counseling session, but in less than ten minutes it was over. "Let God continue to convict you of your judgments and show you more of your wrong attitudes at church and at home. Stop trying to relieve the pressure you're under—let it work for you." I assured them I would take their advice, but privately I was annoyed that they had taken so little time with me. I felt overwhelmed and shocked at what I had just learned about myself. The minister's wife of this large Presbyterian church was full of judgments toward dozens of people in the church. What a lousy Christian I was! Why weren't they more surprised?

Cay and Judy talked about how difficult it was for Christians to be wrong. "Christians don't seem to understand that Christ is the only righteous one," Judy said. "When you see that you are wrong, then you see how much you need Jesus. It is your wrongness that entitles you to a Savior." I had never seen that before. After I had committed my life to God, I thought I could no longer be really wrong about anything. A good Christian was supposed to do everything right, so I kept my ugly thoughts hidden, as if they weren't even there. But invariably, the thought—or a worse one—would come back. I was living in a pretend world.

THOUGHT "" God cannot give us a happiness and peace
apart from Himself, because it is not there.
There is no such thing. ""

(C.S. Lewis, 1898-1963)

Cay and Judy told us that Jesus died for our wrongness. We do not have to work, work, work at being right, but instead we need to flee to Jesus in our wrongness. I didn't know exactly what that meant, but I wanted to find out. I was seeing my need for Jesus Christ as I had not seen it before. When I accepted Christ into my life fourteen years before, I knew that I needed him to change my life and save me from some ugly sins. But I didn't realize, until that week, how much I needed him every day.

God had to be a part of any change that was going to happen in my life, if it was going to last. In Weight Watchers, the lecturer would say, "Before you know it, your tastes will change. You won't want to eat those foods you now love so much." To me, that meant that someday I would not have to even bother to resist; my desires would be gone, and it would all just happen without any more effort on my part. But that day never came for me. I still loved apple pie and chocolate ice cream as much as ever. The self-imposed discipline helped me to achieve my weight goal, but it didn't change my desires at all. And, whenever I cheated on my diet or gained any weight, I would just stay away from the meetings. That way, I didn't have to face my failure.

I had disciplined myself many times before in my life—for a brief period of time and with some sort of goal in mind. But never had I needed or desired the moment-by-moment help of anyone else, including God. My feeling about discipline had been that it was a form of punishment, used only to correct outward behavior. Now I saw the possibility of its being used by God to work a change deep inside me. In fact, not only did I see that possibility, I felt it happening.

At the beginning, I felt as if I were tied up with a thick rope, not able to move without pain. That changed. Instead of my feeling bound, the opposite was happening, and I was feeling free: free from my damnable judgments and my critical attitude toward my husband and my children. I was falling in love anew with my family.

> Instead of my feeling bound, the opposite was happening, and I was feeling free.

the beginning of the THREE D'S

One year after I joined Weight Watchers for the second time, Bill and I rented a cottage on Cape Cod for summer vacation. We had grown to love Rock Harbor, where Cay and Judy lived together with their families and where an intentional community of Christians, known as the Community of Jesus, had grown up around them. And it was on Cape Cod that the first group gathered together to take the teachings of Cay and Judy and put them to use in our daily Christian walk.

Cay Anderson was the first person to put the name "3D" on the process we were all working on. One morning, she laughed and said, "Diet, Discipline, and Discipleship seem like the center of many of the problems that church people have in daily life." Our Christian walk and our daily struggles were disconnected for many of us. We could not figure out how God could or would care about such trivia as dieting. That simple comment from Cay was obviously an anointed thought, because from 1972 until today there has been an unbroken chain of people and groups across the world using the 3D materials.

For some reason this particular vacation time on Cape Cod made me realize that the image of that red "smiley" face in the East Hall at Parkminster Church in Rochester was smiling and encouraging me to take the 3D concept back to our church. I could not stop thinking about it. Could this be God's answer not only for me and for the small group on Cape Cod but also for the many church people at home?

F OR DAYS, I could hardly get my mind off the understanding of those three D's. Bill and I were sitting on the beach one afternoon on Cape Cod, watching the children swim, when for the umpteenth time, I started wondering who back home might be interested in such a group.

"Bill?" "Mm?" he said, absorbed in *Time* magazine. "Do you think Dorcas might be interested, hon?" "Interested in what?" he murmured, not looking up. "Interested in a 3D group back at church." "Maybe." "I bet Margaret and Dee would be, because of their weight problem, don't you?" "Well," he replied, throwing me a quick glance, "I suppose you won't know till you get home and ask them, right?" And he turned back to *Time*.

I knew all he wanted to do was to read in peace, but it didn't seem fair that he should be so peaceful when I was anything but. "I haven't been able to lose ten pounds in the last year, trying by myself," I said.

No answer, not even a grunt. I continued: "I'll bet Norma would love to be involved in a Christian weight group. And Mary Jane is anxious to take off the weight she gained since Kirk was born. That's already five others besides me for a group, and I'll bet Lois would join, too."

"Sounds to me like that group has already started, but you haven't talked to one person yet. What's more, there's no way you can talk to anyone until we get back to Rochester. So why don't you put this whole 3D thing out of your mind and enjoy the last of our vacation. Remember, it will be a whole year before we can get back here," Bill said, putting the magazine over his eyes and settling himself for a snooze.

He was right. It was typical of me to get so wrapped up in something that I forgot everything else. I needed to be thinking about my family and our vacation and not some new program. There would be lots of time for that after Labor Day.

PARKMINSTER CHURCH WAS ALWAYS EXCITING IN SEPTEMBER. It was exhilarating to go over and watch all the activity—the preschool teachers and aides scrubbing and cleaning, the Sunday school staff getting the nursery and the other classrooms ready, and various people painting and cleaning around the church. Fresh home from vacation, I was anxious to check in with the key people who I believed would want to join me in a 3D group.

I recognized Jean's car in the parking lot. She was the program chairman for the women's association and one of the most active women in our church. Jean would be the perfect one to try out 3D on! And just then, as if on cue, she came hurrying out. "Hi, Carol, welcome home!" she said, pausing on her way to her car. "Hope you had a good, restful vacation on Cape Cod." "We did! We enjoyed every minute, as usual."

I could see she was in a hurry, but I didn't want to let her go without at least mentioning 3D. "Jean, I have a great idea for a new program for our women here at Parkminster. I have been thinking a lot about it on Cape Cod this month. And I think it would be a wonderful way to get different people involved." "I'd love to hear about it," she said, opening the door of her car. "Maybe we can get together after the fall luncheon."

After the fall luncheon! My heart sank. That meant October! "I guess I thought it was something we could maybe start soon, like next week . . . and I—" "Oh, Carol," she said, trying to say it kindly, but revealing the pressure she was under, "there's no way I can even think about another program until next spring!"

I should have appreciated all the pressure she was under, but I had one goal, and that was to get some interest in doing a 3D group. "It would be called a 3D—diet, discipline and discipleship—group," I went on hurriedly. "It would be a Christ-oriented counterpart of Weight Watchers. We could use our faith, we could support each other with prayer. . . ." "Carol, please forgive me, but I've got to run. I'm late for a meeting. It's great to have you back again." And she waved, as she got in her car and closed the door.

> It would be a Christ-oriented counterpart of Weight Watchers. We could use our faith, we could support each other with prayer. . . .

Standing there and watching her back out and pull away, I waved, but inside I felt like crying. I tried to tell myself how busy she was, and how unfair it had been of me to grab her and spring 3D on her. But I was also thinking that she had such a good figure and didn't have a weight problem or any lack of self-discipline, so of course she wouldn't be interested.

I tried to remind myself, walking into the church, that if this were indeed God's answer, it would somehow all work out. But not even the smell of fresh paint or the happy bustle of activity could lift my spirits. I started wandering toward the preschool. Then, I heard someone call my name. "Carol? Well, Carol! Welcome home!" It was Dorcas, the wife of our assistant minister. "I saw you talking to Jean outside. Did she tell you that they've sold over a hundred tickets already for the luncheon, and it's still three weeks away? For a supposedly quiet month," Dorcas went on, "August has been absolutely incredible around here. I hope it was quieter for you all at the Cape."

"Well, of course it was quieter, but my mind was extremely busy thinking about a Christian diet program possibility for Parkminster." Now, Dorcas was well aware that I was always thinking about new things at the church, and she knew that every new thing demanded more time and more energy. I loved being a minister's wife, but even more than that I loved creating new ventures. No wonder her first reaction was hesitation!

"Ugh, diet! Don't even mention that word to me—please! I joined Weight Watchers and quit again, just in the month you've been away." She laughed. "I think I'm going to get a pin for being the person who has joined and quit the most in one year." I managed a weak smile.

It was plain to see she was not the least bit interested in any diet group—Christian or otherwise. I didn't say any more, but inside I had the feeling that walls were caving in.

my first 3D GROUP

September began to slip away, day by day. I didn't bring up the subject of 3D again to anyone. I felt so hurt and rejected that I decided that dieting and discipline were just not important enough to bother with. And little by little the needle on the bathroom scale went up, as I enjoyed French fries and ice cream cones whenever I could sneak them in. I was eating and enjoying it, and to heck with every thought of dieting!

But then Lois came to see me.

"Anyone home?" called a voice outside our side door. "Sure," I called out, "come on in."

In walked Lois, bright, cheerful, and excited. "I just wanted to stop by and tell you how well the summer went!" She was beaming. "It's been the best summer we've ever had! That schedule you worked out with me in July was a gift from God to me and my family."

She waited for me to respond. For a minute I couldn't remember what she was talking about, and then it dawned on me. "Oh, I'd almost forgotten about that." I was amazed at her excitement and freedom. She really was different since we had spent a day cleaning and talking about how she could better organize her daily schedule. "Carol, I wonder . . . well, would you mind if I checked in with you on a regular basis, just to keep things going in the right direction?" "Sure, as long as you don't expect me to come and clean every week," I laughed.

The next day, I had another surprise visitor. "Your husband felt I ought to come over and tell you what I just told him," Norma started. "As you know, I've lost a great deal of weight since the beginning of the year, and now I've even started lecturing in the Diet Workshop group I belong to." "I didn't know that you were lecturing, Norma; that's great!" "Well, I'm not sure it's so great. The reason I was able to lose the weight had more to do with my new faith in God than the diet program itself. And that really makes it hard, because I have to sell a diet program—and not talk about God at all." I shook my head in amazement. "Bill tells me you are thinking about starting a diet group based on Christian principles," she continued. "I think it sounds tremendous! I'd love to be a part of it, if possible."

I must have looked surprised. "Thanks, Norma. I did think about that very seriously and then kind of dropped the idea. But it's beginning to seem more possible now." We talked awhile, and I assured her I would get in touch with her when the plans became more concrete.

A few hours later, I had a third unexpected visitor. Ruth walked in, nervously stopping at the top step before coming in the kitchen. "I'm sorry to just drop in this way, but Bill said he thought it would be good if I came over and talked to you. . . ." Then she burst out crying.

"Come in the living room, Ruth, and sit down," I said, putting my arm around her shoulder. Our living room had two love seats; she sat on one, and I sat opposite her on the other. For a few minutes she cried, and I sat there, praying silently. Her crying was coming from so deep inside, it made me hurt. I felt helpless sitting there, but I knew it was good for her just to cry. "I find it really hard to talk to anyone, Carol . . . especially about my personal life. I'm a person who doesn't let people get too close to me." Her voice was shaky and the crying continued in between pauses. "All I want to do lately is sleep. The minute Dan leaves for work and the children go to school, I go back to bed and sleep half the morning away. Then, believe it or not, I go back to bed after lunch and sleep half the afternoon. I just don't want to be with anyone or do anything." She started crying hard again. "The minute people begin to get close to me, I pull away."

"What can I do to help, Ruth?" I asked. "I don't know if anyone can help me," she sobbed. "I'm running from my responsibilities, and I'm running from my friends, and I'm running from God. I have such a good husband in Dan, and three children and a beautiful home—so much to be thankful for. But I'm so unhappy with myself!" It was clear that she hated herself for showing such uncontrolled emotions. "Ruth, I want to help you. And for heaven's sake, don't feel embarrassed about crying," I said, feebly.

Ruth and Dan were newcomers to the church. She had always been friendly to me and was an enjoyable person to be around. I remembered the lovely lunch she had had, the day I had gotten to know Lois. Ruth had been the perfect hostess, making us feel at ease, and her home was beautiful and decorated tastefully. Like Lois, Ruth was a teacher and did substitute work at the same school. She had been concerned about the project Lois had taken on at school and how involved it had become. I remember having the distinct feeling that Ruth really cared about Lois and me. I had never dreamed she was so unhappy inside. But thinking about Lois reminded me of the good results Lois had had with a daily schedule. Maybe Ruth could use help with her schedule as well.

"Ruth, ah, have you ever tried to specifically plan your days hour by hour?" I asked sheepishly. "You mean some sort of a daily schedule?" she replied. I was surprised she even had any idea what I was talking about. "Yes, that's exactly what I mean," I said. "If you planned your day with certain things at specific times, you might be less tempted to go back to bed." "Lois was telling me how much she had been helped by her new schedule," Ruth remarked. "And I can see a big change in her attitude and her feelings about her house and family."

I couldn't help wondering, as Ruth talked, how a schedule would work out for her. She seemed to be able to keep a beautiful house and still have time for creativity—like flower arranging and needlepoint and things that added special touches to her home. But as she talked, her needs became more apparent. "I started making draperies and a bedspread for our bedroom two years ago, and they're not finished yet. And I have several other projects started, but not finished. I'd also like to get to know some women from church better, and I thought it would be fun to have a few small luncheons—I love to cook and entertain. But if I don't break this habit of running off to sleep every chance I get, none of those things can get done." She seemed to relax as we talked. Her eyes were puffy, red, and swollen from crying, but she was also at ease.

"I'm sure I look awful, but I feel better," she said, as she was getting ready to leave. "Thanks a lot—I'll need help to set up my schedule. Can we get together to work on it soon?" She went on, "Will it be all right if I call or stop in before the weekend? I want to start a new way of living Monday morning," she said with a big smile. "Sure, Ruth," I said, wondering when I was going to get the time in my own schedule to work on someone else's. I had Lois checking in with me, and now Ruth—who would be next?

I had mixed emotions when Ruth drove out of the driveway. Where would I find time for all of this? I decided I shouldn't worry about it. God would have to stretch my days, that was all there was to it.

That night at supper Bill asked how my day had gone. I laughed and said, "Not on schedule, that's for sure." Then I told him about my morning visitors. "Sounds to me like God is answering our prayers about whether there should be a diet, discipline, and discipleship group here," he laughed. "He sure seems to be making it obvious." "Well," I replied, "let's quickly tell the Lord I'm willing, before I have ten more women coming one by one, asking to be put on schedules."

That very night I called Lois, Ruth, and Norma and shared the 3D idea with them. They thought it sounded tremendous and could think of several other women who would be interested in a group like this. So we set up a meeting time—the next Tuesday night at eight o'clock in the church lounge.

TUESDAY NIGHT ARRIVED—and so did ten women! I had invited Dee to come. She was a very heavy woman, a Catholic, who had phoned me one afternoon in reference to something I had written in my column in the local newspaper. I had talked with her several times since then and knew she had a big weight problem. She needed help and was delighted that I had asked her to come to our meeting, even though she didn't know anyone there but me.

Then Lois had asked Margaret, who was in choir with her, and Mary Jane if they'd be interested. They were; both weighed over 200 pounds (90 kilos). Mary Jane had lost a lot of weight a few years back, but then gained it back again during a pregnancy.

The heavier women were obviously wondering why in the world Jo and Beverly were in the room. Neither of them weighed more than 120 pounds (55 kilos). I had asked them to come, not because they needed a diet group, but because I felt they could help us get some direction.

They were both very active in Christian groups in the community with their husbands and seemed to lead very disciplined lives.

Then there was Norma, looking great from her dieting. Helen came, too. She had been in the Weight Watchers' group Dorcas and I had been part of, and like us, she had dropped out. And Dorcas reluctantly agreed to come too.

There was an uncomfortable silence in the room. I knew I had to get the meeting started, even though I didn't have the slightest idea what we were going to do. "I guess I should start off." I shared my ups and downs with the 3D idea: I wanted it desperately because of my own weight problem, and yet I had not been willing to step out on faith to begin. "I'm ready now, with God's help, to see just what he has for us. Certainly, if the secular world can offer so much help to the overindulger, God has to have an even better answer. More and more I am seeing, and I think others are too, that our lives are totally undisciplined."

> More and more I am seeing, and I think others are too, that our lives are totally undisciplined.

At this point, Lois jumped in. "This summer Carol helped me get myself on a daily schedule, with specific times to clean each room in my house, do my laundry, and even play the piano and hike with the kids. We took a totally disorganized life, rearranged things with God's help, and it has completely changed my life in less than two months." She was radiant, sharing the blessings of the summer with the group.

Mary Jane talked about how defeated she was, having gained all her weight back during her pregnancy. "I need help," she said, rather desperately. She was an attractive woman in her late twenties, but her weight was an obvious burden to her.

Norma spoke of her frustration with not being able to talk about God in her lectures at the diet group.

Jo and Beverly, the two who I thought would be able to guide us, confessed a lack of self-discipline in many areas of their lives. "Just because I'm not heavy doesn't mean I'm a disciplined person," Jo said. "I need help in a lot of ways." Beverly wholeheartedly concurred, and Ruth openly shared her struggle with sleeping too much.

We all agreed that we needed God's help and each other's help.

"Well," I announced, "here we are: the fat, the sleepy, and the sloppy, without a choice between us!" And we all roared with laughter. We all agreed that we needed God's help and each other's help, and so we decided to meet every Tuesday night at eight, and just see what would happen.

Someone suggested we pray before we leave. Spontaneously we stood up and joined hands in a circle. A spirit of quietness came over the room. An hour or so before, we had not known each other's inner struggles, but now, through sharing, we were becoming closer. God had been in our midst, and we all knew it.

THOUGHT 66 Common sense and good nature will do a lot to make the pilgrimage of life not too difficult. 99

(Somerset Maugham, 1874-1965)

By our fourth meeting, we realized that our group needed a leader. "Where in the world have you been?" Bill asked me drowsily, squinting at the clock. "Is that twenty minutes of twelve?" Once again, I had come home late after a 3D group meeting. I wished I hadn't bothered to turn on the light to get ready for bed. "I've been at the 3D meeting over at church," I replied, heading to the bathroom. "Four hours at a 3D meeting? That doesn't sound very much like discipline to me!"

He was right. The next week, I wasn't the only one to mention that we were sometimes wandering aimlessly in our conversations. Helen and Ruth, too, were concerned about the same thing. And then Margaret spoke up. "You know, we might as well face it: what we really need for the group is a leader."

"I agree," Dee chimed in. "And the other problem we have," Ruth stated, "is that no one wants to really speak up. I didn't get the help I needed last week, and I didn't help anyone else, I'm afraid. And what good is a group like that?" she asked bluntly.

"How about you, Dorcas?" I asked. "You're a teacher and a good one; you could do a great job." "You've got to be kidding! Me, the big flunky from every weight-watching group in town, leading a diet group? It will be a major accomplishment for me just to stay in this group until the end of the program." She laughed. And then everyone else laughed with her, and that broke the tension.

Someone suggested we pray about who should lead. A great idea, I thought; why hadn't it occurred to me?

But before we could pray, Lois said, "Carol, as the senior minister's wife, aren't you the most likely one to lead the group?"

"Lois," I replied, so vehemently that I startled myself, as well as the others, "I'm tired of leading groups! Let someone else lead for a change." The tenseness returned to the room, and I knew it was my fault. My attitude was dreadful. Feeling a little sheepish about it, I said, "I guess we'd better ask God to help us to know his will about this."

So we prayed together. After that prayer time, the way seemed very clear. The group asked me to lead, and I was pleased to say yes. Dorcas said she was also willing to lead, if need be, and this meant her heart had been changed too. So Dorcas and I decided to try to lead the group as a team of two. This way, there would be an added check and balance, as two hearts were often better at hearing the Holy Spirit than one.

Dual leadership was also being tried all around us, both in public school education and in Sunday school. That sounded terrific to me. So, in spite of our discouragement and resistance as a group, God moved us on. The leaders were ready, the group was enthusiastic, and we were all aware of God's presence and direction in a new way.

We decided that our meetings should last only one hour. We would all weigh in before meeting time and start right at eight. And we agreed to pray for each member of the group every day. Mary Jane volunteered to type up a prayer list for us with names and telephone numbers. We felt like a real group now, venturing together on a new path.

Once we began to seek God's will for our 3D group, and set guidelines of discipline for ourselves, I felt excited and happy as Tuesday evenings approached. I even looked forward to leading the group, and I sensed that much of the change in my attitude was directly attributable to the daily prayer—both mine for all the others in the group, and theirs for me.

But our mutual commitment had turned out to be a lot harder than any of us expected; it was also producing unexpected results. None of us had had very much practice in laying aside our own cares and concerns in order to fully concentrate on the needs of others, even for only a few minutes a day. But we were beginning to get the hang of it.

At first, I resented the prospect of coming to know the other women's failures. I felt my own were enough for me to cope with! I did not want the responsibility of having to care about others, too. But I soon became deeply convicted of what an ugly attitude that was—it was about as far from Christ's as it was possible to get. And never mind spiritualizing it; I knew plenty of non-Christians who cared more about other people than I did. I was sorry. I determined to care enough to take the group members' needs to God, and that was the very best care I could give.

GOD DID NOT EXPECT ME TO HEAL THEIR WEAKNESSES or carry their burdens. But he did expect me to listen carefully and then take their needs to him. And what's more, the other members were doing the same thing with my needs. We were all part of a team, working together, to get our lives more under the control of God. It was not a chore but a privilege.

We were learning a great deal in a hurry—not points of doctrine, but practical ways to put our faith in God to work in the most mundane things of daily life. It became more and more apparent to me that my Christianity revolved almost entirely around me, rather than around Christ. Oh, of course, I brought the big things of my life to him. But the little things—the shopping list, the order of the day's priorities—were still my domain. I did things my way and in my time, and God had very little to do with them. And yet I knew from the Bible that every hair on my head is numbered, and that not a sparrow falls to the ground without the Father in heaven being aware of it. I had always accepted those facts in my head, but I had no idea how to translate them into my life.

Now I was beginning to see that if God cared about the sparrow's fall, he would be interested in my shopping list. The small, personal concerns of my life and the greatness of God's love were finally coming together. The smallest, most insignificant details of my daily life were opportunities to glorify him. Imagine eating, working, sewing, cooking, and cleaning house to the glory of God! Along with this new awareness, I was now becoming convicted of my disobedience in little things. The still, small voice that I had successfully ignored so many times by telling myself that God couldn't possibly care about such small details, was becoming louder and clearer all the time. He did care—I was the one who didn't.

As the whole idea of doing even the littlest things to the glory of God became clearer for me, I began to see why I had been so uncomfortable in my previous diet group. The emphasis of that group

> The whole idea of doing even the littlest things to the glory of God became clearer for me.

had been to help me become a better me! I dieted so I could wear nicer clothes, get more attention from my husband and family, and have a good self-image. I was at the center, but the center of my life was supposed to be God.

The old way had worked. I felt a hundred percent better, I bought new clothes, my husband loved the new me, and people at church and everywhere else raved about how wonderful I looked. But where did God fit into all of it? He didn't! I had been on an ego trip—a self-glorifying experience that, if I was interested in drawing closer to God, was exactly what I did *not* need.

Instead, I was beginning to realize that diet is not about what I eat or don't eat so much as it is about my whole life! Now, more than 35 years after that first 3D group began, I invite you to join with me in this new venture, *Your Whole Life*, combining expertise from Maggie Davis and the wisdom that for three and a half decades has sustained 3D groups all over the world.

getting YOUR OWN GROUP STARTED

If you feel the way I felt back in 1973 and believe that this concept is what you have been looking for, we would like to give you a few tips about starting a group in your community. We encourage you to register on our website, www.3DYourWholeLife.com, and then access a variety of free resources available to 3D Group Leaders. Guidelines for leading a 3D Group are in the appendix of this book and also online in downloadable PDF format. In addition, you'll find discussion questions online for each of the twelve weeks; answers to the most common questions about foods, nutrition, eating behaviors, and disordered eating; and guidance on when to refer a group member to a professional.

3D GROUP MEMBERS

■ Meet for one hour, once per week, for twelve weeks

■ Keep a daily food journal

■ Memorize a verse of Scripture each week

■ Read the devotionals and the Scriptures each day

■ Weigh in weekly

■ Pray for each member of your group every day

■ Share the ups and downs of your weekly journey.

your whole life

Weeks 1–12

The Plan

EATING RIGHT

- Fill out the Initial and Quarterly Health Assessment.

- Determine your Body Mass Index and Health Risk.

- Use the *Your Whole Life Journal* daily.

LIVING WELL

- Use a pedometer to determine how many steps you take in an average day.

- Put a fresh flower or a nice plant on your kitchen table this week.

LOVING GOD

- Read your daily devotions, and memorize your Scripture verse.

- Pray for five people every day.

God Has the Answer

I OFTEN HEAR THIS QUESTION: Why a "faith-based" diet program? Or even, what does "faith" have to do with dieting?

My quest in the early days of this journey was to learn how to apply the faith I had in God—the faith that believed he could move mountains and that he kept my life in balance—and apply it to my daily struggles. Each of us struggles; my struggles were primarily with my weight, my self-image, and my self-worth. I wanted to take my spiritual beliefs and put them to work in my daily life. Surely that was possible.

The revolving door of fad diets, weight loss, and weight regain had consumed much of my young adulthood. That is why I want to assure you from my own experience: if you have been dieting on and off for most of your life, you need to know that you have not failed at diets. Diets *have failed you.*

I knew beyond any doubt that God cared about everything I was concerned about. The Bible says that he cares about sparrows, and even about the hair on your head! So why wouldn't God care about my struggles with eating? While asking that question, I looked up at a Sunday school bulletin board and a simple sign that read, "God Has the Answer." I knew then and there that I had to incorporate God fully and completely into the nitty-gritty details of my daily life.

> Does God have answers? Yes, he does.

Does God have answers? Yes, he does. He has answers for all of our needs. We just have to learn how to listen, and believe. That's your first challenge as you go forward with the 3D plan this week!

Don't rush this process, even if you want to start losing weight *right now*! We encourage you to take twelve weeks to read this book. Again, don't rush this process, or the likelihood of success will diminish. Nowhere is slowing down more necessary than in the sections at the end of each week—the daily devotions.

If the changes in your diet and lifestyle are to be permanent, they must become part of your whole life, each week and each day. Remember this: those who monitor themselves while trying to make changes have a greater chance of losing weight, while those who do not monitor themselves at all while undertaking changes may actually gain weight in the long run.

The fact that you have picked up this book and have started reading it tells me you are already feeling that you want to make a change in your life. For you, the program has already begun. Your heart is ready, and results will start happening.

Here's what you need to do to get started: Look in the back of this book for the "Commitment Card." Fill it out, keep the top portion for yourself, and then send the bottom part back to the 3D office. This is an important and necessary step. You are the only one who can decide what changes you need to make in your life. Then let *Your Whole Life* guide you over the next twelve weeks.

Your Whole Life IN MOTION

Exercise therapist Ed Haver taught me twenty years ago how important it is to get moving, regardless of how much time you have to devote to it. Take a few minutes at this early stage in the program to answer a few questions. Discuss your answers with others who are supporting you in this process.

- Do you usually exercise?
- How often?_____
- With what intensity?_____
- Does a certain time of day seem good for you to consider exercise? What time?_____
- What type of exercise do you think you would do?_____
- Would you consider wearing a pedometer to help you get a better understanding of your daily movements?_____
- Do you belong to an exercise program or a health club?_____
- Starting today, how many minutes of exercise could you realistically commit to, daily, for the next twelve weeks?_____

Making Choices

I recently saw a popular magazine at the supermarket checkout counter with a cover photo of an oversized, mouth-watering frosted layer cake on a pedestal. The featured story in small letters beneath it read something like "Lose 15 pounds in 15 days!" This is typical of the mixed messages we see in the media. We are encouraged to think that we can have our cake all the time and be thin, too!

Most diet and weight management programs begin with giving "dieting" advice in the first session or the first chapter. The fact is that most individuals want and expect to lose ten to twenty pounds quickly after starting a program. **It's no accident that weight loss program marketing often promises unbelievable weight loss or includes unrealistic claims or exaggerated results that are not sustainable over time.**

The responsibility is yours to make your own choices, and not have them imposed on you. Over and over I see clients who have tried liquid diets, diet pills, fad diets, and special foods. Those who blindly follow what someone else has prescribed for them will sooner or later fail, because they are not learning about why they eat what they do and how to change eating and exercise habits for their whole life.

While we will show you how to estimate how many Calories[1] you need on an average day, and how much of various kinds of foods you may want to include in your daily diet, we urge you to place the emphasis on what foods you need to increase in your diet, rather than just on foods to reduce or eliminate. Once you start to eat better you may find it easier to avoid or decrease portions of foods that aren't as nutritious.

You need to draw on your inner strength and values to determine whether that scrumptious cake or a healthy body is more important to you. And perhaps you can find a way to have a small portion of a sweet in the context of a generally healthy diet. Our intention is to help you find a lifestyle that will meet your individual needs and address your unique food issues. This is not a restrictive diet, but rather a process of getting to know yourself better, and learning to make better food choices in the context of your whole life.

So we ask you to be patient and to reflect on your motivations and expectations for eating right. Devote some time this week to assessing your own weight, body mass index, health status, risk factors, and other important personal health considerations. Before you start on this journey to eating right you need to know where you are starting, so turn now to the Appendices of this book and fill out the *Initial and Quarterly Health Assessment*. You will start the journey to eating right as you complete this first step toward knowing yourself better. (You may need to obtain some of this information from your physician.)

You can use this information in the chapters/weeks ahead to decide on your motivations and to set your goals, and you will use this information to determine what action steps you will need to take. We will ask you to reassess these

questions at the end of the twelve-week program, and every three months from then on.

Contributing Factors to Weight Gain

Portion choices are a major contributing factor in weight gain, but there are other factors as well. Genetics are something we can't change, but they are a major internal factor in weight gain. You may also be taking essential medication that contributes to your gaining weight. These are environmental and external factors. So are your eating behaviors and lifestyle habits. It has often been said that genetics (your family health traits) load the gun, and your environment (your diet and exercise) pulls the trigger. Your lifestyle habits can also cause your metabolism to slow down, as happens with yo-yo dieting. (Visit www.3DYourWholeLife.com to download a Your Weight History questionnaire. Your answers will help you not only to determine where you are now, but also to identify clues from past efforts that can help you with 3D.)

We do know that a weight loss of as little as seven to ten percent of your total body weight can bring a significant reduction in health risk. Look in the Appendices at the Body Mass Index Chart and find your Body Mass Index (BMI). BMI is a way of using your height and weight to identify your risk and to track your progress as you make changes. BMI is roughly a way to determine the percent of a person's body fat, and it works well in most cases, with the exception of those who are quite fit and those who are quite out of shape.

Tips for Men

Although more women than men are responsible for putting dinner on the table, the fact is that children generally model their eating more after what dad eats than mom. Since the average man prefers to eat corn or peas and not a wider variety of vegetables, this means that many children aren't exposed to a bigger variety of foods. Children may need as many as fifteen to twenty exposures to a new food to even decide if they like it or not. Even adults may need repeated tastes of new foods to develop a taste for them. Think of wine-tasting and how wine connoisseurs develop a palate that can appreciate the subtle differences in flavor of many types of wine. You may not like plain boiled and mashed squash, but you may love it roasted with olive oil and drizzled with balsamic vinegar. So give vegetables a second look, and give your children the legacy of a wider acceptance of foods. Try a new vegetable on the grill next time you cook out. Keep an open mind, have an adventurous palate, and try to keep to yourself any negative comments about a food that you don't like; let others decide for themselves if they like a particular food.

Current research is underway to examine the role of these internal and external factors and to seek treatments that will make a lasting difference in preventing and treating weight gain. In the meantime, we must look to achieve a balance between Calories consumed to Calories burned, and to the inclusion of healthier food in the diet.

It is important to become aware of what and when you are eating. This week you should start to keep a record of what you are eating. (Purchase *Your Whole Life Journal*, which is designed for this purpose— see the back of this book for details— or use the simple online Food Record, available at www.3DYourWholeLife. com.) Start this week by writing down what you are eating, with an amount or a description of the foods eaten.

You may find it helpful to draw a line after you finish recording a meal or a snack so that you can look back and easily analyze specific meals and the pattern of your eating throughout the day. Identifying what you eat at specific times in your journal entries can help you see a pattern (or lack of one) in your daily eating. Although you should begin recording your diet in your journal each day, the decisions to eat right are actually made meal by meal. So don't be overwhelmed by looking at a whole day. Just have faith that if you don't make the best choice at one meal, the next meal or snack is another opportunity to make a better selection.

Your Risk of Health Problems Increases as Your Weight Increases		
BMI less than 25	Normal Risk
BMI 25–30	Increased Risk
BMI 30–35	High Risk
BMI 35–40	Very High Risk
BMI 40 or more	Extremely High Risk

Maggie Davis

using a PEDOMETER

Use a pedometer to determine how many steps you take in an average day. This exercise is help you gain self-awareness for this first week. Keep a record of the number of steps you take each day, and at the end of the week, total the steps and divide the total by seven. Now you know your average number of steps per day. (You can order a pedometer online at www.3DYourWholeLife.com or from the 3D office.)

If you haven't already done so,
please consider forming your own group,
so that you don't go through this program by yourself.
Invite four or five friends from your community
or your church to join you on the journey.

Have them call 3D at 1-800-451-5006 or visit
www.3DYourWholeLife.com
to get what they need to join you.

Week 1 Daily Devotionals

Theme for the Week FAITH

Verse to Memorize *Be still, and know that I am God.*

—PSALM 46:10A

Day 1   "I Am the Lord Your God"

READ | Exodus 20:1–6

I am the LORD your God, who brought you out of the land of Egypt, out of the house of bondage. (v. 2)

The theme for this week is *faith*. What this really means is that we must begin these reflections by talking about God, because the central element of our faith is not ourselves but rather the One in whom our faith is placed.

We are tempted to think that believing is primarily something *we* do and that, therefore, we are either good at it or not so good at it. Like the muscles of our bodies our faith is then either weak or strong, depending on how "heavy" the circumstances are that we are facing. "I haven't much faith these days," we say in times of trouble; or, "I'm not sure I believe that God can do this," we say in the face of seeming impossibilities. These are perfectly legitimate admissions, and they sometimes describe exactly how we are feeling. But notice the first word in these sentences: *I*. Should the existence and meaning of faith really begin with me?

The people of Israel came to know and believe in the God of Abraham, Isaac, and Jacob not because they sought him out but because he introduced himself to them—"I am the Lord your God." Every experience of God's power working on their behalf was like their re-introduction to the Lord of the universe. Their faith became rooted in *God's* strength, *God's* love, *God's* promise.

Before we offer our faith to God, God offers *his* faithfulness to us. Before it is a bold confession, faith is a grateful response. Again and again God introduces himself to us. Faith is simply our confident answer: "*You* are the Lord my God."

REFLECT | *What is the greatest and most loving thing God has done for you? Consider the events of recent days—where can you now recognize God's presence or power? Tell him what it means to you for him to be in your life.*

Day 2   Jesus Is Lord

READ | Acts 16:22–34

"Men, what must I do to be saved?" And they said, "Believe in the Lord Jesus, and you will be saved. . . ." (vv. 30–31)

The word slips too easily from our tongues: "Lord!" But when Paul and Silas answered the Philippian jailer's desperate plea, directing him to believe in "the Lord Jesus," this was no glib instruction. The word *kurios* had a very particular meaning in that day. It was the term used to address the Roman emperor, the sovereign and supreme monarch over all the land. The word meant "authority and power," and it was the duty of all citizens to respect and obey their *Lord.*

But this is precisely where difficulty arises for the Christian soul. How glad we are to welcome Jesus as Savior and Redeemer. He comes to us in our need, binds up our wounds, comforts our sorrows, and pardons us by his own sacrificial death on the cross. Anyone who has found this glorious freedom of forgiveness knows that words can never fully describe the depth of what that experience means. Where we run into trouble, however, is in translating that genuine sense of indebtedness for the Savior's love into daily obedience to him as our Lord. This is where our faith is put to work.

Having faith—*believing* in the Lord Jesus Christ—has very practical implications. Jesus said: "Not everyone who says to me, 'Lord, Lord,' shall enter the kingdom of heaven, but he who does the will of my Father who is in heaven" (Matthew 7:21).

REFLECT | *Try to describe one of your own experiences of Jesus' forgiveness and love. What does it mean for Jesus to be Lord over your whole life?*

Day 3   Lord of All

READ | Mark 4:35–41

Who then is this, that even wind and sea obey him? (v. 41)

The disciples marveled that, simply at the sound of Jesus' command, the roiling seas became calm and the swirling winds ceased. At his word the storm was stilled. It should not be any surprise to us that Jesus' word is greater than all the forces of nature, for it is by his will that all things exist in the first place. Heaven knows for certain what we believe by faith: "In the beginning was the Word. . . . He was in the beginning with God; all things were made through him, and without him was not anything made that was made" (John 1:1–3).

We, too, are part of his creation, and this makes Jesus Christ the Lord and Ruler of *my* universe. As I move about this day, I look to see him at work—to see the expression of his will and wisdom in the ordinary as well as the extraordinary. Not only in the stormy sea, but in the rustling grass, in the songs of birds, the passing of clouds and sunshine, I look to see the signs of his creative and providential hand. I, and the world in which I live each day, exist under the sovereign oversight of God.

There were those in the Gospels whose unbelief prevented Jesus from doing mighty works among them (Matthew 13:58). As close as they were to Jesus, they did not recognize him for who he truly was. For this reason, let us not set a limit on what God can do. As you begin this course of discipline, set your aim high. Listen for his command, and keep your eyes on him who is Lord of all.

REFLECT | *Take a few moments today to reflect on the mystery of just one item of God's creation. What lessons does it offer about Jesus' lordship in your own life? What are those places in your own "universe" where you do not recognize Jesus as Lord?*

Day 4   Lord of the Ordinary

READ | 1 Kings 20:26–30

Because the Syrians have said, "The LORD is a god of the hills but he is not a god of the valleys," therefore I will give all this great multitude into your hand, and you shall know that I am the LORD. (v. 28b)

The Syrians made a big mistake in thinking that God was not in the valley! Apparently they respected his power on the hills, but thought they could get away with whatever they chose when it came to fighting in the valleys. This limited scope in their vision would prove to be their undoing.

Let us take the valley, in this case, to speak of the commonplace, the ordinary, the familiar. Here, surrounded by hillsides and shadows, there are no grand vistas, no broad and distant horizons. The valley presents no unknown territories to be conquered—just the common, the everyday, the usual. How easy it is to lose our larger vision in such places, to forget what we saw when our hearts were brightened on the mountaintop of inspiration. In the valley the vision fades and we return to reality.

But "reality" is exactly where we encounter God. Was it not in such places that Jesus met the people he came to save? They were walking the streets, sitting at supper, praying in the synagogue, working in the fields, drawing water from wells. These "valleys" became the actual meeting places between heaven and earth.

In the weeks ahead, we, too, need to meet Jesus in our "valleys." We need to know him in the ordinary places of our lives—the mundane tasks, the familiar relationships, the normal worries and concerns and hopes that make up our everyday lives. After all, he is already there, for he is the God of the valleys as well as the hills.

REFLECT | *Where have you already discovered Jesus' presence in your daily routine? What ordinary tasks do you face where you need to know that Jesus is Lord?*

Day 5 Lord of the Mountains

READ | Isaiah 49:8–13

And I will make all my mountains a way. (v. 11a)

We sometimes speak of "mountaintop experiences" to describe times of brilliant inspiration or ecstatic joy. The Scriptures are filled with examples of such encounters between God and his people: Mount Sinai, the Mount of Transfiguration, Mount Zion. But there are other kinds of "mountains" as well, mountains that speak to us of what is impossible or impassible: the mountain of Abraham's testing (Genesis 22), the Mount of Olives, the mount of Calvary. These are the mountains of trial, and there is no way to ignore their looming presence in our lives.

But stop and think! The mountain you face, which appears so hard to climb, is the Lord's mountain. "I will make all *my* mountains a way," says the Lord. Whatever the difficult circumstances in your life at this moment, God in his great mercy and love for you has made them *his* circumstances. If the obstacles were yours alone to face, you would have reason to feel discouraged. But these mountains are not yours alone. God already stands upon them as Lord.

Although you may long for greater ease, less demanding tasks, a more level road, this mountain way you walk is God's appointed path for your healing and salvation. Not only has God set you upon it, but he promises to be with you every step of the way. Yes, the way can be hard, even dreary. But keep your eyes up! Keep moving. The heavenly company is cheering you on, and Jesus himself, "the pioneer and perfecter of our faith" (Hebrews 12:1–2), supplies you with sufficient strength to take each step. The truth is that we need the mountain way, for no other way leads to the fulfillment and fullness of life that Jesus offers.

REFLECT | *What testimony do you have already of God's presence in and provision in an "impossible" situation? What "mountain" do you face today?*

Day 6   Lord of Our Relationships

R E A D | Colossians 3:12–16

If one has a complaint against another, forgiving each other; as the Lord has forgiven you, so you also must forgive. (v. 13)

Jesus taught us to pray, "Forgive us our trespasses [or sins] as we forgive those who trespass [or sin] against us." This is the acid test of our prayer's sincerity before a holy and all-seeing God, "before whom all hearts are open, and from whom no secrets are hid" (in the words of a traditional prayer for "purity of heart"). Every time we pray the Lord's Prayer we ask God to forgive us in the same way that we have forgiven others. A frightening thought indeed, especially when we consider what is secreted away in the recesses of our own hearts!

Many of us have learned to hide our negative and unforgiving feelings toward others. We feel guilty about having such thoughts and feelings, and so we conceal them, even from our own scrutiny. After a while, we may even have a hard time remembering what the hurt or offense was in the first place. But forgetting does not necessarily mean forgiving, for there it still lies, buried away and unresolved, unless, from that same heart, we truly forgive.

Our buried resentments, often going back to the early days of our lives, can be the unconscious source of many difficulties—including the way we feel about ourselves and the way we feel about others. Only the Holy Spirit, the "Spirit of truth," can unearth that which we have so carefully buried away, and bring it out into the light so that genuine forgiveness and healing can take place.

Ask the Spirit of Truth to reveal those hidden wounds and resentments that take up space in your own heart, so that you can bring them to the Cross of Jesus. There, in the presence of a Love that has laid down his life for your forgiveness, do not refuse to forgive those who have hurt and wronged you. This is an essential part of what it means for Jesus to be Lord of your relationships.

R E F L E C T | *Make a list of the people who have influenced your life. Ask yourself the question, "Do I hold anything against anyone on this list?"*

Day 7   Lord of Our Minds

READ | 2 Corinthians 10:1–6

We destroy arguments and every proud obstacle to the knowledge of God, and take every thought captive to obey Christ. (v. 5)

Who is in charge of the thoughts that fill your day, the secret things that pepper your mind? Is Jesus Christ the Lord of your thought life?

The saints have known forever that the mind is the battleground where Satan does battle against the children of God. He uses every subtlety, every temptation, every vain imagination he can muster in order to lure and distract God's children from the path of faith and obedience. He especially uses our sense of right and wrong—our self-righteousness and our guilt. On the one hand, his object is to keep us from facing and admitting our wrongness because he does not want us to know the cleansing and freeing power of God's forgiveness. On the other hand, he means to condemn us for our sin, so that the weight of guilt in our hearts will weaken and paralyze our faith.

If in our thoughts we harbor anger, jealousy, resentment, and the like, we will eventually act according to those thoughts. Likewise, if we are harassed by fear and guilt, we will fail to make faithful decisions as we seek God's ways for our lives. Jesus himself said that it is the things in our hearts that dictate the actions of our lives (Mark 7:21). This is why our innermost thoughts must be brought to kneel before their Lord. They must be at *his* service.

Jesus wants to be the Lord of the thoughts that rule our minds. Let him begin to point them out to you, and then submit them to him through confession and repentance. Do not despair when the battle for who is in charge of your mind begins to take place. As ancient Christians used to say, the devil does not bother with those who are already thinking according to his ways. The fact that there is a battle at all means that you are beginning to "bring your thoughts captive to Christ" who is Lord even of your mind.

REFLECT | *What thoughts do you find to be the most distracting for you? What are those ways of thinking that most quickly undermine your faith in God?*

The Plan

EATING RIGHT

▨ Continue to keep a daily food journal of everything you eat and drink. Determine how many servings of fruits and vegetables you eat each day.

▨ Plan what you are going to eat for breakfast and lunch every day this week, and prepare in advance to avoid impulsive eating.

LIVING WELL

▨ Keep track of your daily steps, and see if you can add more steps this week. There are easy ways to add steps: park your car farther away from the store, take the stairs instead of the elevator or escalator, or get up to change the TV channel instead of using the remote control.

▨ Plan to read a magazine and look for fun tips to help you "live well" this week.

LOVING GOD

▨ Read your daily devotions, and memorize your Scripture verse. Repeat your memory verse every day, out loud if possible.

Discipline
and Preparedness

DURING THIS WEEK, WE WILL FACE THAT WORD—*discipline*—and we will begin to take that word that has so many negative and threatening connotations and turn it into a positive, faith-building word. Know that if you begin to submit yourself, in these weeks in front of you, to specific spiritual and diet disciplines, there will be wonderful benefits.

A Bible verse to memorize is Hebrews 12:11: "For the moment all discipline seems painful rather than pleasant; later it yields the peaceful fruit of righteousness to those who have been trained by it." Please write this verse on a piece of paper and tape it to your bathroom mirror. Believe God's answer about the area of discipline. Remember: Just the simple practice of memorizing one verse each week could be life-changing.

Another important challenge for this week has to do with being aware of your daily activity that will or will not burn Calories. I am a busy person, and I have been shocked to know how many days each week I would be classified as sedentary just because I spend so much time at my desk, in my car, or at the sink or stove. Think about *activity* this week instead of food. You've read or heard that we should walk up stairs instead of taking the elevator, or park farther away in the parking lot so that we have to increase our steps. Let's actually do these things this week. Instead of asking your children to take out the trash, do it yourself, just for the exercise. Carry in the groceries or mow the lawn. Make a conscious effort to walk more steps this week than you did last week.

You are being equipped this week; you are becoming more whole, and moving is part of the process.

> You are being equipped this week; you are becoming more whole.

THOUGHT   ❝ Search out our hearts and make us true,

Wishful to give to all their due;

From love of pleasure, lure of gold,

From sins which make the heart grow cold,

Wean us and train us with thy rod;

Teach us to know our faults, O God. ❞

(William Boyd Carpenter, 1841–1918)

Replacing Old Habits

Discipline is a word that often evokes negative feelings and can make us feel like naughty children. The term *discipline* is derived from the Latin word for "pupil" or "student." But discipline and punishment may be synonymous in your mind. In relation to finding a healthier way of eating, discipline refers to replacing old habits with new ones. Discipline can mean proactively including healthy foods that form the foundation of healthy eating. Discipline may mean planning what you will have for dinner tonight. It may even mean that you will not skip meals or that you will always eat your meals at the table.

Discipline also involves work; it is not necessarily easy. Your menu will not be dictated by someone else. Instead, you will need to take responsibility to plan meals that work for you. That way, you will learn to establish a method for eating right rather than going on and off a diet. You can start simply by modifying the type and amount of food you are eating now.

If you prefer using a structured meal plan, here are two easy ways of selecting a Calorie level to start the process.

1) You may already know how many Calories you need each day. You may have had your metabolism checked by your healthcare provider, your health club, or a personal trainer. If so, use that number and round up to the next closest Calorie level.

2) If you don't know your metabolic rate or the specific Calories you need, you can use the chart below as a rough guideline for the Calorie intake to target:

If you weigh in pounds (kilos):	Target Calorie Level
less than 150 (68)	1200
150–199 (68–90)	1400
200–249 (91–112)	1600
250–299 (113–135)	1800
300–349 (136–158)	2000
350–399 (159–181)	2200
more than 400 (182)	2400

You can use these Calorie levels and the Recommended Daily Portion Guidelines found in the Appendices first as a way to determine if you are eating enough vegetables and fruits. We'll refer again to these guidelines later in the book.

Many people find that they need to learn new ways of discipline to replace outdated, nonproductive ways of eating that they have practiced consciously or unconsciously for years. We ask you to start this process where you are right now. You don't have to change everything you eat or throw out most of the food in your refrigerator and start over. If you're like most people reading this book, you also have a family to feed and to consider in these changes.

Preparing healthy food daily and exercising daily are both sacred work. This is work that no one else can do for you. If you are using this book as part of a group program, you will have the help and support along the way of others who are also striving to eat right. You may even arrange to trade off the preparation of meals with a friend or a neighbor. You may decide that some days, the best you can do is to stop at the supermarket for a cooked chicken and a salad to go. Look at the journal you kept this week. Start to note the types of foods you are eating. Think about the times of your meals and snacks. Take a few minutes each morning to map out what you plan to eat that day. Even if unexpected changes occur, you will be prepared to eat right. These small steps can lead to big changes in your eating. Think of this journey as a marathon, not a short sprint. Marathon runners don't start training by running all 26 miles at once. They start slowly and add incremental changes in their routine. You are gradually, day by day, meal by meal, building habits for a lifelong journey.

Eating Right with Habits and Portions

One of the first things I suggest to my clients is that if they aren't eating breakfast, they should begin eating at least one small item or snack such as a piece of fruit or a small piece of whole grain toast. Eat something in the morning to break your fast. There is scientific evidence that eating four to six times per day can help with weight management. So, if you're skipping breakfast or eating only two meals per day, your first goal might simply be to eat three meals per day.

Now, before you get scared, let me explain what I mean by a meal or a snack. A meal can be two or more foods from different groups. It could be a spoonful of peanut butter on a whole grain cracker with an apple for a meal on the go, or it could be a soup with vegetables, chicken, and beans for lunch. For breakfast, it might be a biscuit of shredded wheat, a handful of berries, and some nonfat or low-fat milk. A snack might be a small portion of one or two food items.

ten-percent weight loss will reduce your health risks.

Whatever goal for weight loss you have in mind at the outset of the program, we recommend you divide that in half, and then you may have a realistic weight loss goal. Above all, focus on goals that involve specific lifestyle habits, such as planning your meals in advance, preparing food ahead, being aware of impulsive eating, making conscious decisions about portions, and so on.

Setting Goals

Remember that all goals need to be positive, practical, and maintainable. We recommend that most goals be directed first at habits and portions. If you are setting a weight-loss goal, start slowly (e.g., five to ten pounds) and then reset your goal when you reach that level. A reasonable weight loss goal is to lose one-half to two pounds per week. Those with more to lose may find that they lose more at first than those who have only a relatively small amount of weight to lose. A goal of a seven- to

Maggie Davis

Good Lunch Habits

Lunch is often an accidental meal for those who are eating away from home at school or work. There are few topics more important for discussion in your group than the discipline of lunch preparation. Leaving home without a prepared lunch involves risk. If you are ordering out, you may be dependent on where and what co-workers want for lunch. Do you depend on drive-through fast food? Will you even take time for an actual lunch break? Why not try packing a lunch once a week? Take a brown bag, an insulated tote, or a lunch pail with a simple sandwich, a piece of fruit, some nuts, and some raw vegetables. Or pack your lunch the night before with leftover items from dinner. You may even find that this habit will ease the temptation to have second helpings.

Maggie Davis

Week 2 Daily Devotionals

Theme for the Week DISCIPLINE

Verse to Memorize *For the moment*
all discipline seems painful
rather than pleasant;
later it yields the
peaceful fruit of righteousness
to those who have been
trained by it.
—HEBREWS 12:11

Day 1 Under the Lord's Training

READ | Hebrews 12:1–11

For the moment all discipline seems painful; . . . later it yields the peaceful fruit of righteousness to those who have been trained by it. (v. 11)

To those who have been trained by it: What does it mean to be under the Lord's training, to undergo discipline for the sake of learning his ways? We have already reflected on the truth that Jesus is the Lord of every aspect of our lives and that placing our faith in him means acknowledging his supreme reign over all. This includes all of the words and circumstances that enter our lives. For example, we have the choice, in response to anything that is said to us or that happens to us, either to allow Jesus to use it for our good, or to throw it away like some useless scrap.

Pressure and even pain can make our hearts hard and bitter, or they can break the hard shells of our hearts and make us soft and merciful. The outcome depends on whether or not we will allow ourselves to be trained by what comes our way. Even a word of correction spoken by a husband, wife, parent, employer, or friend either can cause anger and resentment, or it can motivate us

to humble ourselves and to change. If we let a word of correction work in our favor—which means letting God use it in our lives—then we can be "trained" in the Lord's ways by anything that comes our way . . . *anything.*

The choice is ours. The athlete who strives to win must undergo painful exercise and rigorous discipline to get into shape. The musician preparing for concert-quality performance must give many hours to diligent practice, day after day. The soldier preparing for battle must submit to relentless discipline and training. Sometimes the regimen can be very difficult. But it must be embraced if the goal is to be achieved.

As disciples in the service of our Lord, we cannot afford to be soft on ourselves if we want to live like Jesus, to the glory of God. We cannot afford to be undisciplined children, living by every desire and feeling of the moment if we want to grow to be mature men and women of Christ. The goal is well worth the effort. The discipline may not be pleasant at the moment, but keep your eye on the goal—and on the Leader. He has already endured his discipline!

REFLECT | *What pressures are in your life right now that God intends to be instruments in your Christian training? How can you better cooperate with God so that they can be useful disciplines?*

Day 2   The Fruit of Suffering

READ | Romans 5:1–11

More than that, let us rejoice in our sufferings, knowing that suffering produces endurance, and endurance produces character, and character produces hope, and hope does not disappoint us. . . . (vv. 3–5a)

Christianity does not glorify suffering or praise suffering for its own sake. Jesus says to his followers, "I will not leave you desolate" (John 14:18), "Peace I leave with you" (John 14:27), and "These things I have spoken to you, that my joy may be in you, and that your joy may be full" (John 15:11). Joy, not suffering, is the keynote of his life, and even the suffering he underwent was for the sake of "the joy that was set before him" (Hebrews 12:2). Is there a clue here to what Paul means when he exhorts his readers to rejoice in their sufferings?

First, we can rejoice, knowing that God can use even suffering for our good and that our pain does not have to go to waste. The Cross itself is the prime example of this mystery. Life comes out of death, joy comes out of mourning, strength comes out of weakness—this is a sure and certain promise for those who follow Christ.

Second, we can rejoice in experiencing the presence of Jesus in ways in which we cannot know him when everything is bright and pleasant. Stars can be seen only at night, and many hidden things of God can be received only in and through the darkness of our suffering. As we endure the things that cause us pain, we come to know our Lord in a deeper and more intimate way.

Finally, we can rejoice, as did Jesus, because in the kingdom of God suffering is not allowed to have the last word. The Cross was not an easy thing for Jesus to bear. The Gospels make this truth painfully apparent. Neither is our own cross an easy thing for us.

Through the suffering of Christ, God brought about his kingdom on earth. Through our own suffering, he brings that kingdom into our own hearts. Endurance, character, hope, even joy—these are signs of the kingdom of God, and they are the fruit of suffering in the name of Jesus.

REFLECT | *How can you cooperate with God so that he can turn suffering into a blessing in your life? What thoughts and feelings can diminish the constructive value of suffering and turn it into a destructive experience?*

Day 3   Add to Your Faith

READ | 2 Peter 1:1–11

If these things are yours and abound, they keep you from being ineffective or unfruitful in the knowledge of our Lord Jesus Christ. (v. 8)

Salvation is a free gift! We come to the Lord in our helplessness and need, and he saves us by his own grace and through the sacrifice of his own life on the cross. This stands forever as the great, unfathomable mystery of our faith. It is the eternal Good News. Catherine Hankey's familiar gospel song says it well:

> I love to tell the story,
> 'Twill be my theme in glory
> To tell the old, old story
> Of Jesus and his love.

This good news of Jesus and his love remains the touchstone against which everything else must be measured. Our hope and our salvation lie in who he is and what he has done for us.

The apostle, however, gives us an important reminder that even in the joyful knowledge of Christ's grace and love we may become ineffective and unfruitful—unless we do *our* part. Even though Jesus has paid the full price of our redemption, we are enlisted to add our own efforts to the mix, to be "co-laborers" in God's field. Paul referred to himself, and to us, as "God's fellow workers." Therefore, the Scriptures challenge us to "add to our faith."

The list of qualities we are to add is impressive, even staggering: virtue, knowledge, self-control, steadfastness, godliness, brotherly affection, and love. It shows us where the inner battles are to be fought and where our work as Christian men and women truly lies—for most of us have far to go before achieving all these traits.

Let God speak to you about where you need to pay closer attention to one or more of these areas in your life. Do not let disappointment in yourself or discouragement rob you of eventual victory. The list might be long, but so too is the strong arm of our Savior, and he has promised to be our help and salvation.

REFLECT | *Which item on this list of "additions" do you find most challenging? How can you pursue it?*

Day 4   Discipline—the Love of the Father

READ | Deuteronomy 8:5–16

Know then in your heart that, as a man disciplines his son, the LORD your God disciplines you. (v. 5)

The generations of Israel were taught to see God's love and instruction as the chief defining realities of their lives. "He declares his word to Jacob," sings the psalmist, "his statutes and ordinances to Israel. He has not dealt thus with any other nation" (Psalm 147:19–20a). From the time of Abraham, the Lord had set his love upon this people, all the while knowing full well that they would be a rebellious house: "Sons have I reared and brought up, but they have rebelled against me. The ox knows its owner, and the ass its master's crib; but Israel does not know, my people does not understand" (Isaiah 1:2b–3).

Yet God never ceased his love for them!

In the passage from Deuteronomy, we are reminded of the forty-year wilderness experience Israel underwent before reaching the Promised Land. They were being led out of bondage by the mighty hand of God. But the route of escape took them "through the great and terrible wilderness, with its fiery serpents and scorpions and thirsty ground where there was no water. . . ." And the reason for all this was "that he might humble you and test [or prove] you, to do you good in the end" (vv. 15–16). The hardships they endured were meant to strengthen and purify them, to forge them into an instrument of God's blessing in the world. God's discipline *was* God's love. Ask any parent and he or she will tell you that, for the sake of the child, the two qualities are inseparable.

It is a simple fact of human nature: without discipline we become like sheep without a shepherd, wandering aimlessly through the hills, interested only in the next thing that attracts our attention or will please us. We grow lax and presumptuous, eventually taking God's love and grace for granted. But, under the loving discipline of God, we are led to the greenest pastures. We grow into mature sons and daughters who enjoy a loving relationship with the Father, knowing their own need of his discipline and the amazing love that lies behind it. For through his discipline, God's loving purpose is "to do you good in the end."

REFLECT | *How do you come to know that God's discipline is his love? Today, where do you see God's fatherly discipline in your life?*

Day 5   Your Share in the Fight

READ | 2 Timothy 2:1–11
Share in suffering as a good soldier of Christ Jesus. (v. 3)

Take your share. What is your share of suffering? Does it seem that you have been allotted *more* than your fair share? Have you ever wondered if the martyrs facing the deadly beasts of the Coliseum thought they were being asked to endure more suffering than was reasonable? Or, what of those human torches whom the wicked emperor Nero set afire and used to light up the roads leading to Rome? Or, what of the soldiers in the Battle of Hastings, or at Valley Forge, in the swamps of Vietnam, or in the deserts of Iraq? Take *your* share, says the apostle Paul! To follow Jesus Christ is to enter into a spiritual battleground. We know this to be true simply by reading the Gospels. And we know it to be true by our own experience. Therefore we ought not be surprised when we encounter suffering.

As "good soldiers" of Christ Jesus, we are enlisted under the banner of the Cross. We have heard his call in our hearts and we have received the amazing love and forgiveness he offered to us in our need. Now he says, "Behold, I send you . . ." and we find ourselves plunged into a war that has been going on since the time of Adam and Eve. It is the most crucial battle of all history, and it cannot be won by those who surrender to self-pity, self-indulgence, or self-justifying rationalizations. Our daily disciplines are battles to be fought and won, side by side with our fellow soldiers and under the command of our Lord. It is certain that there will be more battles ahead, and we must be ready to face them. But final victory is equally certain, for Jesus Christ has risen from the dead! So, do not be afraid. *Take your share.* "Be watchful, stand firm in your faith, be courageous, be strong." These words from 1 Corinthians 16:13 inspired Isaac Watts to write this:

Must I be carried to the skies
On flowery beds of ease,
While others fought to win the prize
And sailed through bloody seas!
No! I must fight if I would reign!
Increase my courage, Lord.
I'll bear the cross, endure the pain,
Supported by thy Word.

REFLECT | *What spiritual battles do you face this week? What are the hindrances in your life that keep you from victory?*

Day 6 Take True Aim

READ | 1 Timothy 6:11–16

Fight the good fight of the faith; take hold of the eternal life to which you were called when you made the good confession in the presence of many witnesses. (v. 12)

In this passage, young Timothy is urged to "aim at righteousness, godliness, faith, love, steadfastness, gentleness" (v. 11). His older and wiser mentor, the apostle Paul, certainly knew that Timothy would not always hit the target, but still he charged his spiritual protégé to keep on aiming!

There is no place for discouragement and no valid reason for it in the Christian life. Yes, we are prone to discouragement, and we all experience it. In its most acute forms it can be debilitating. You may even be experiencing it today. But learn to recognize it for what it is—the symptom of a more critical malady, a sign that you have lost sight of some basic truths. For, when we get discouraged, it is because we have put too much faith in ourselves and too little faith in Jesus. We have underestimated the seriousness of our condition and presumed too much upon our own strengths and abilities. We have forgotten how

radical a change following Jesus truly requires. When we fail—and failures are as inevitable to our human condition as the setting sun is to day's end—we give way to discouragement because it is easier to surrender to disappointment than it is to renew the fight. We are our own worst enemies.

So, away with discouragement! Eternal life, says Paul—life in all its fullness, peace, and contentment—is ours by the gift of God's grace in Jesus Christ. This includes all of the strength we need to follow Jesus faithfully to the end. Therefore the apostle charges us to constantly "lay hold" or "take hold" of that life. This means fighting the good fight, fully engaged in the battle against "the world, the flesh, and the devil." Remember, discouragement is one of the devil's chief weapons. But discouragement can be defeated by one of the chief weapons in our own arsenal—the truth. We overcome discouragement by recalling for ourselves the truth about who we are and the truth about who Jesus is. So, take aim—take true aim—at the things of God's kingdom. And do not lose heart.

REFLECT | *Are there areas in your life where you would rather give in to discouragement than to "fight the good fight"? What are they? If you have been discouraged about anything this week, how did you handle it?*

Day 7   Are You Ready?

READ | Matthew 25:1–13

But the wise took flasks of oil with their lamps. (v. 4)

What has discipline to do with vigilance? Jesus' parable of the wise and foolish maidens makes the connection for us. A state of readiness requires that all be in order, that priorities be straight, and that vision be clear. It means looking beyond the needs and wants of the moment, and remaining alert for whatever may come our way. Only discipline—learning and conforming to the ways of God— can prepare us for an unknown future. As we do our best to fight against self-love, self-indulgence, and carelessness, we "tune up" our souls for the challenges and tasks that lie before us. But, if we are negligent in our prayers, our reading of God's Word, and our personal habits and obligations, we are like soldiers who are not prepared for the call to battle. The enemy will surely come and find us unaware!

The Lord, too, bids us to be ready for "his appearing," not only at the hour of his coming again, but at the hour of death and, in the meantime, at whatever hour he may seek to enter the door of our hearts. Are we in a state of readiness for him? This does not mean frantically looking around at every moment, or living anxiously for the future. The discipline of readiness means "having our house in order," living faithfully in the "now," and doing wholeheartedly whatever God sets before us to do.

There is a lesson for us in the legend of the crane. In the monastic tradition, the crane has been considered a symbol of vigilance and order because of the story of its watchfulness. According to legend, the cranes would gather each night and select one among their number to keep watch through the darkness. To ensure that it remained attentive, the guardian crane would balance itself on one leg, and hold a rock in the upraised claw of the other. Then, if by chance it fell asleep, the rock would naturally drop upon its foot and awaken it. This is a state of readiness that certainly requires discipline!

The crane and the wise virgins: both are examples for us of what it means to stand at the ready, even during the darkest and hardest hours, always prepared for the coming of the Lord.

REFLECT | *What personal disciplines are weakest in your own life? What can you do to begin to strengthen them?*

THOUGHT 66 We only need to focus on God with our will. That's all. It's our choice, and because God loves us, we can do this. 99

(Teresa of Avila, 1515–1582)

Week 3 Will Power— Yours or God's?

The Plan

EATING RIGHT

▪ Examine your journal. Look at your meal and snack pattern so that you will become aware of people, places, and thoughts that influence your eating.

▪ Substitute one whole grain food for a refined carbohydrate you usually eat.

▪ When you shop, look for whole grain products, such as whole grain English muffins, as alternatives to highly refined foods.

LIVING WELL

▪ Is your pedometer count moving up each week? What is your average number of daily steps? Can you increase this daily by 200 steps?

▪ This week, think about organization. What does it mean to you? What works in your household, and what doesn't? What is the cause of your clutter, and what could you do about it? What items are essential? What items are most important to you?

LOVING GOD

▪ Sometimes we need a change of scenery in order to pray. As Emilie Griffin writes in *Doors Into Prayer*, "Going to a different place, or perhaps an uncluttered space, clears the decks and focuses our concentration. Perhaps also we need privacy, and a sense of safety, in order to open up to God entirely." This week, find a new place to read your devotions and pray.

Will Power—
Yours or God's?

RIGHT NOW YOU ARE ENTHUSIASTIC, you are encouraged, you have a new book in your hands. You feel excited about what God can do in the practical areas in your life. That's exactly how you *should* feel!

But the fresh feeling of what's new will not take you the whole way. You need to discover—and probably rediscover—what will power is all about.

This is the week to start focusing on your will power. There is a difference between determination and will power used for their own purposes, and will power that leans on God. You need to bring discipline into your life, and do it now, but you need to do so while resting completely in God's arms. He will help you throughout the day.

God uses will power to touch us, strengthen us, and push us. You will be reading about these things in this week's devotions, and I hope that this week you will recognize daily when you are leaning on God and when you are leaning on yourself. Be attentive to this.

In these first few weeks, give it all you have! Give all the will power you have to follow the direction and the guidance in this book. And then, expect God to honor that commitment.

The Scripture verse to learn for this week is Luke 22:42: "Nevertheless not my will, but thine, be done."

Gradual Changes for Permanent Results

I often hear my clients say, "I don't have any will power." What they may actually be thinking is, "I can't starve myself for more than a few days." If you have repeatedly tried severely restrictive and unbalanced diets for a week or two and found that you couldn't continue to eat that way for very long—you, too, may equate that experience with a lack of will power. So, what is will power? Will power starts with a goal and a plan. It is fired with motivation and action and courage. Learning to eat right and live well takes motivation, courage, and overcoming inertia by taking action.

How do you know you're ready to change? Well, since you're reading this book that tells me that you are consciously thinking about changing the way you eat. You must be ready to be patient at this point to avoid being overly restrictive. If you go "cold turkey" you may lose those 15 pounds in 15 days, but you are bound to fail in the end and regain even more weight than you lost.

The Balance of a Healthy Diet

A healthy diet should provide enough protein, energy (otherwise known as Calories), water, vitamins, minerals, antioxidants, and phytonutrients to meet the needs of an individual in his or her particular stage of life. Your eating plan should include the following essential whole foods:

- Whole fruits
- Vegetables
- Whole grains
- Lean, high-protein foods (fish, poultry, meat, soy, eggs, beans, nuts)
- High calcium foods (dairy, soy)
- Highly unsaturated oils and fats
- Supplements as needed

Most of us do not eat enough fruits, whole grains, or vegetables, so that is the category we need to focus the most attention on in the beginning. Once you include these basic foods, then you can add other foods for interest, taste, and variety.

In addition to selecting healthy foods, examine your daily Journal and look at your meal and snack pattern.

Ask yourself these questions:

- Are most of my Calories consumed at dinner?
- How many times a day do I eat?
- Do I eat differently depending on where I am and who I am with?

Remember the objective: You want to establish new habits, not go on a temporary diet. It is important, for instance, to increase your intake of fruits and vegetables slowly to let your body adapt to the changes. Do you remember the TV ad that declared, "You can't fool Mother Nature"? Well, your digestion needs to adapt to an increase in fiber content!

Next, examine how your intake compares to the other food groups. You might decide to try to increase one portion per day of one or two of the food groups. These foods can help you displace some of the overly refined and low nutritional value foods you may have been eating.

Maggie Davis

Week 3 Daily Devotionals

Theme for the Week THE WILL

Verse to Memorize *Nevertheless not my will,*
but thine, be done.

—LUKE 22:42

Day 1 Thy Will Be Done

READ | John 5:30–44

I seek not my own will but the will of him who sent me. (v. 30b)

Long before Jesus was born, the psalmist prophetically spoke of him by the Spirit, saying, "Lo, I come; in the roll of the book it is written of me; I delight to do thy will, O my God; thy law is within my heart" (Psalm 40:7–8). Of Jesus it could be said, and of no other, "His will was in perfect harmony with the Father's will." This is what Jesus is saying in the Gospel passage for today's reading. Confronted by those who are challenging his authority to teach and to heal, Jesus freely admits that the sole purpose of his coming is to do the will of the One who sent him. He is not looking to promote his own authority or to exert his own will upon others. He can teach us to pray to our Father, "Thy will be done," because his whole life is a fervent offering of that selfsame prayer.

This does not mean, however, that Jesus was never tempted to divert from God's will. Though sinless, he nevertheless was fully human, and therefore subject to the same temptations encountered by all men and women, from the time of Adam and Eve. Persuaded by the lies and seductions of God's enemy (and ours), our biblical forebears rejected the will of their Creator for the sake of having their own way. But Jesus Christ, the new Adam, resisted the temptations of the devil by committing himself completely to God's truth. He kept his will in undivided oneness with his Father. "Although he was a Son," says the writer to the Hebrews, Jesus himself "learned obedience through what he suffered" (Hebrews 5:8).

Since the Lord and Savior of all mankind has fully tasted the bitterness of temptation as well as the sweetness of victory, we would be foolish not to listen to his teachings in this matter, or not to follow his example. Who is in a better place than he to come alongside us in our own pursuit of God's will? Who is in a better position than he to assist us when we begin to weaken in our resolve, or even when we fall? Every day he sought out and accomplished the will of his Father. Can we not trust him, then, to help us seek and do that same divine will? "Father, thy will be done."

REFLECT | *There is a wise saying that goes like this: "I can't stop the birds from flying over my head, but I can stop them from nesting in my hair." How can this be applied to the experience of temptation? What does it mean to "nip temptation in the bud"?*

Day 2   "Teach Me to Do Thy Will"

READ | Psalm 143

Teach me to do thy will, for thou art my God! Let thy good spirit lead me on a level path! (v. 10)

Clearly, the psalmist wrote these words amidst circumstances of deep trouble and turmoil. The seriousness of his plight is almost palpable in the language he uses to describe it: *I am crushed . . . to the ground; my spirit faints within me; he has made me sit in darkness; my soul thirsts . . . like a parched land.* In such a situation of suffering, we all know how appealing it is to wallow in the mire of self-pity and to think dark, vindictive thoughts against our "enemies." In fact, some of the psalms are very candid in expressing that kind of grief and anger. And they help us to find language for our prayers when our own language fails us. God seems to be saying, through the Psalms, that it is all right

to recognize and express these deep emotions to God! After all, he knows that we are feeling them better than we know it ourselves.

But there is more to this poem than the author's complaint. "I have fled to thee for refuge!" writes the psalmist. The place to flee in the midst of our struggles is to God, the only secure place of refuge. God is the only place of hope and comfort and safety. However, this is not only a peaceful place; it is not only a resting place. And it is most certainly not a place where we will be patted on the head and told simply that everything will be all right.

The very next verse tells us that it is also a place to learn: "Teach me to do thy will, for thou art my God!" To remain in the place of refuge, and to know the peace we all long to have inwardly, we must seek to know and to do the will of God. Running to God in our troubles is the beginning of their solution. The rest comes when we ask him what he wants us to do.

"For my thoughts are not your thoughts, neither are your ways my ways, says the LORD" (Isaiah 55:8). Because this is so, we need to be taught his ways and his will. He teaches us his will in many ways, and even though we may not find his disciplines easy, there is tremendous fulfillment in following them. We are learning as we follow. Our prayer is being answered even as we pray.

REFLECT | *What complaints or griefs do you have to bring to God? What is he teaching you about the next steps he wants you to take?*

Day 3   Saying and Doing

READ | Matthew 21:23–32
Which of the two did the will of his father? (v. 31a)

All four Gospel writers tell us that, after entering the city of Jerusalem for the last time (today's passage describes events on the day after Palm Sunday), Jesus was questioned again and again by the religious authorities. From every angle his enemies scrutinized his words and his behavior, essentially asking him, "What gives you the right to say and do such things?" It was in answer to these charges that Jesus spoke about the meaning of true obedience by telling the parable of the two sons. Above all else, Jesus' concern was for his accusers to know "which of the two did the will of his father?"

We all know that it is easier to move our lips than to move our lives. The promises we make with our voices cost us little until we are required to follow through with our actions. Saying and doing can be quite different things altogether.

Sometimes we meet the word of God to us—be it through the instrument of others or of circumstances—with such a force of resistance and upheaval in our hearts that the first word out of our mouths is, "No! I do not want this! I will not do this!" After a time, however, and by the grace of God, we begin to consider the foolish or even defiant stance we have taken. Our resistance begins to weaken, and we begin to feel bad for setting ourselves so fiercely against doing God's will. We may pray. We may even shed tears of repentance. But the most important thing is that we begin to see how wrong we are, that we have no right to say no to God. Eventually, like the first son in Jesus' story, we turn around and do what God has required of us. We may not like it. We may not enjoy doing it. But we do it anyway!

On the other hand, in the second son, Jesus describes a most dangerous spiritual condition—the self-deception that can lurk in the human soul. The second son was pleasant and agreeable, readily agreeing to do his father's bidding. Because he did not outwardly oppose his father, he may even have counted himself to be a good and obedient son. Certainly most of us have done something similar, and it may take us some time to realize that we never did the thing we agreed to do. We are not as obedient as we think we are. Jesus is saying here that more than lip service, more than promises, more than "I go, sir," are required. Sooner or later, we must *do* the will of the Father. Better sooner than later. Better now than tomorrow. Better deeds than words.

REFLECT | *In what ways are you like either (or both) of these two sons? What has God asked you to do for which you need to give him an answer today?*

Day 4   *Becoming* God's Will

READ | Mark 1:16–20

Follow me and I will make you become fishers of men. (v. 17)

As Christians, we live between what we have been and what we are yet to become. Our lives are in the process of being changed by the re-creative hand of God. It may seem at times like a particular area of our lives will never be different, never improve. But we have the declaration made by

Jesus to his followers—"I will make you become. . . ." It is a certainty that, if we will follow, we will be changed. We are *becoming*.

So, what is it that we are becoming? The result depends on the aim and direction of our hearts. Jesus said, "Follow me," meaning therefore that the prerequisite for being remade by God is to follow his Son. If our hearts are "toward the Lord," if we are truly seeking his will for our lives, then the change made within us, however slow and painful it may be, is moving us toward conformity to the likeness of Jesus. However, if our hearts are stubbornly set upon doing our own will, following our own course, then what we become over time will most certainly not be more like Christ. Consider older people, for example, and you can see that they show in clearer, less hidden ways what they have been becoming for many decades. They can be encouraging examples to us of the fruit of obedience to God, or their lives may serve as a warning to us not to choose similar ways.

The Gospel tells us that it is not God's will that any should perish, but that all should come to eternal life. His will is life-abundant, for all. This should help us to remember that doing the will of God is meant to be the pathway to blessing and fulfillment. "For my yoke is easy, and my burden is light," Jesus said (Matthew 11:30). The gospel of Jesus Christ is not some new legalistic program for making our way to a holy God. The good news is the promise that we can learn to "walk by the Spirit," being guided both by inward impulse and by outward circumstances, with the help and fellowship of others, along a path of life. It is a path of *life*, a movement from where we have been to where we are going. At times we are discouraged; at other times, we are exalted and full of joy. But, because we keep on following we keep on *becoming*, seeking more and more to "do the will of our Father in heaven." Let this truth penetrate your thoughts and flood you with new zeal and hope!

REFLECT | *Where can you already see that your life is changing because you are following Jesus? Where specifically is Jesus inviting you to follow him today?*

Day 5 Are You Willing?

READ | John 7:14–31

If any man's will is to do his will, he shall know whether the teaching is from God or whether I am speaking on my own authority. (v. 17)

The world has always resounded with scores of voices calling for the allegiance of the human heart. The "noise" can be deafening. Our current generation is no different and may, in fact, be worse. With all the different doctrines, ideas, and teachings confronting us, it is no wonder that people feel confused. Maybe you are one who has felt this confusion. Perhaps you have asked yourself the question, "How can I know? How can I be sure?" In this passage we hear Jesus saying that there is a definite connection between our willingness to do God's will and our ability to know truth from falsehood. Unless there is in us a deep, underlying desire to find and do the will of God, we can be tossed about by all kinds of half-truths, quarter-truths, or downright falsehoods. Look at the evidence all around us.

This does not mean that we always like doing God's will, or that we always succeed in carrying it out. Paul is a good example of this. As we know from the New Testament, he gave up everything to follow Christ, he suffered many hardships—he was beaten, stoned, shipwrecked, rejected—and endured many disappointments. Yet, writing from prison, he says, "Not that I have already obtained this [goal] or am already perfect; but I press on to make it my own . . ." (Philippians 3:12a). His will was set to move forward with his Lord.

This is the foundation upon which is built our entire knowledge of God and his ways. If we want to know his truth and power in our lives, we must fix our wills firmly in place—like the rudder of a ship set upon a steady course—to do his will. When, however, our hearts are divided and our wills are unruly, when wanting God's will is mixed with what is really a preference for our own, the result will always be confusion and uncertainty.

Tempting as all other voices might sound (including and especially our own!) we must not allow them to distract us from God's appointed path for us. In his instruction for community life, Benedict of Nursia (sixth century) wrote: "What, dear brothers, is more delightful than the voice of the Lord calling to us? See how the Lord in his love shows us the way of life" (*Rule of Benedict*, Prologue).

REFLECT | *Think about an area of your life where you are feeling confused or uncertain. In what ways do you perhaps not want God's will in that area? Try to be as honest as possible.*

Day 6   When the Will is Defective

READ | Romans 7:13–25

I can will what is right, but I cannot do it. (v. 18b)

Has the condition described here by the apostle Paul ever been your experience? The question is rhetorical, for I am sure that you will readily admit, along with me, that you have known the frustration of this conflict more times than you can count. One important thing this malady reveals to us is that there is much about our human soul that we do not understand. Even science will tell us that we often act out of hidden, unrecognized motivations that lie deeply buried within us. It has been the sobering experience of Christians in all ages that we can desire what is good, but that we cannot always accomplish it. Our own strength is not enough to do God's will on earth as perfectly as it is done in heaven. We may want to do it, but in actual experience, there is still too much of the old earthly nature alive in us. We are not yet sanctified, mature, and whole in Christ.

Paul essentially says that all Christians know times when they live under the holy rule of Jesus as well as times when they live by and give expression to this "old nature." One commentator on these verses writes that there is no believer, however advanced in holiness, who cannot adopt the language used here by the apostle: "Everyone feels that he cannot do the things he would, yet is sensible that he is guilty for not doing them. Let any man test his power by the requirement to love God perfectly at all times. Alas! How entire our inability! Yet how deep our self-loathing and self-condemnation!"[2]

Confronted with the defectiveness of our wills, we must turn for help to God in hopeful prayer and to others in honest disclosure. By sharing our weakness and faults, by exposing to others the spiritual blemishes that we would rather hide from sight, we bring before God's healing light those things that would otherwise remain festering in the shadows. We give our brothers and sisters in Christ permission to be our aides, speaking to us God's curative truth and helping us in our struggle to do God's will. As parts of a larger Body we come to know God's grace through the ministry of our fellow members. Thanks be to God for his merciful provision!

REFLECT | *To whom can you admit and expose your needs? Why is it hard to do this?*

Day 7   Living by the Will of God

READ | 1 Peter 4:1–19

Arm yourselves . . . so as to live for the rest of the time in the flesh no longer by human passions but by the will of God. (v. 1b–2) Therefore let those who suffer according to God's will do right and entrust their souls to a faithful creator. (v. 19)

I heard a certain preacher once say that, when he was a child, the only time he heard about "the will of God" was when someone died. People would stand around and say in hushed voices, "It was God's will." As a result, said the preacher, when he became a man and someone happened to mention "the will of God," he would think to himself, "Has it come to that?"

How many of us think that God's will is generally associated with what is hard or unfair or painful? How many of us, when we struggle with the question of our own wills versus God's will, actually believe that all God wants is whatever costs us the most? The one-talent man in Jesus' parable said accusatively to his master, "Master, I knew you to be a hard man, reaping where you did not sow, and gathering where you did not winnow; so I was afraid . . ." (Matthew 25:24–25). Too often, when we strive for what we know God does not want, we hurl the same kind of accusations at God—consciously or unconsciously. And then we work to rationalize our desires and to make his will conform to ours.

If we insist too long and too hard, God may give us up to our own wills. He may simply let us have what we are demanding. The Scriptures tell us of just such occasions. But God is not obligated to make things turn out the way we think they should or hope they would. If we insist on our own way, we may have to live with the consequences.

Yes, living by the will of God may be a real struggle—it is for most of us. But he promises that in his will we will be cared for and blessed. We may not have all the details just the way we want them, but we will find that our wants and his will can more and more become one. Has making your choices according your "passions"—according to what *you* desire or demand—really brought you freedom and peace? Has fearfully (and accusatively) avoiding God's will really brought you happiness? Why not then choose to live by his will?

REFLECT | *Where have you found that giving up your own will in favor of God's will has resulted in blessing? Where have you experienced disappointment or even pain in getting your own way?*

THOUGHT 　　**❝** He speaks, and list'ning to his voice
New life the dead receive,
The mournful broken hearts rejoice,
The humble poor believe.
Hear him, ye deaf; his praise, ye dumb,
Your loosened tongues employ;
Ye blind, behold your Saviour come,
And leap, ye lame, for joy! **❞**

(Charles Wesley 1707–1788)

Week 4 Learn to Listen

The Plan

EATING RIGHT

- Listen to your body's signals for hunger and fullness, and record them in your daily journal. Can you tell the difference between food hunger and thirst?

- Try eating part of your lunch and then wait for 15 minutes to see if you are satisfied rather than completely full. Eat the rest later in the afternoon if you need a snack.

- Carry a nonperishable snack with you in case you can't have a regular meal; an example of this is 1 ounce (30 grams) of nuts and 6–8 apricot halves. Keep these kinds of snacks at work, as well.

LIVING WELL

- Do you realize that housework burns Calories and adds steps to your pedometer? Make your daily responsibilities part of your "living well" category this week, and keep counting your steps.

- Get outside for a walk or a drive at least three times this week.

LOVING GOD

- Add three more people to your prayer list.

Be still, and know that I am God.
Psalm 46:10a

W E MAY HEAR, BUT ARE WE ACTUALLY LISTENING? I learned very early in my marriage that although my husband could recite word for word what I had just said, he was *not* listening. He was watching the Red Sox, doing a crossword puzzle, and letting me talk. He had and still has a great capacity to do many things at once with his mind. But over and over again I found him either not remembering what I had said or not doing what I had asked. (Now, if he were writing this book he could tell you my own sin of not listening!) There is so much to learn about food and health and exercise, and I have heard so many spiritual truths from speakers and books, that I always need to be sure I am really listening. I must pause and prepare my mind and my heart to listen and to expect to hear new things from God. Listening, then, requires me to make new decisions in my daily life.

You are now starting your fourth week, and you need to focus on listening. Voices come at us from many different directions asking us to listen. Advertisers, friends offering advice, advertisers once again!—all try and persuade us to do things. These many voices can be confusing, and they can easily take us off track. But then there is the inner voice of God. How in the world can we discern that still, small voice amidst the noise of our lives? With concentrated effort and a determined will we can listen and we will hear.

That is our focus for this week: to listen for God's voice. Ask yourself these three questions: Are you eating right? Are you living well? Are you loving God? After you ask yourself those questions, be still and listen, and write down specific answers.

In your daily devotional readings, listen for God's voice. Underline sentences and keywords and return to them throughout each day. God speaks to each of us about different areas of our lives. We do not all hear the same convicting words in each reading. What is God saying to you? Use the wisdom of the daily readings, and the quotes from classic sources throughout this book, to encourage you and sharpen your listening for the Holy Spirit. The Scripture verse for memorizing this week is from Proverbs 1: "But he who listens to me will dwell secure and will be at ease, without dread of evil" (v. 33). What a promise! If I listen I will be secure and at ease and without dread.

THOUGHT **❝Tell God all that is in your heart** as you would to a dear friend. Tell him your troubles, that he may comfort you; tell him your joys, that he may sober them; tell him your longings, that he may purify them; tell him your dislikes, that he may help you conquer them. Talk to him of your temptations, that he may shield you from them; show him the wounds of your heart, that he may heal them; lay bare your indifference to good, your depraved tastes for evil, your instability. Tell him how self-love makes you unjust to others, how vanity tempts you to be insincere, how pride disguises you to yourself and others. If you pour out your weaknesses, needs, troubles, there will be no lack of what to say. You will never exhaust the subject. It is continually being renewed. People who have no secrets from each other never want for subject of conversation. Blessed are they who attain to such familiar, unreserved intercourse with God. ❞

(François Fénelon, 1651–1715)

Hunger and Fullness

Physical hunger is a primal instinct. It can't and shouldn't be ignored for very long. If hunger becomes significant and you delay eating for an extended period of time, you may find yourself overcompensating when you eat next. For some individuals, skipping meals may actually trigger a binge. You may eat more quickly due to extreme hunger and your body's urgent need to eat. You may eat too quickly for your brain to get the signal that you've eaten enough, and then find yourself too full later. In other words, extreme hunger may lead to losing control.

Eating somewhat more often may actually be a way of preventing overeating.

It's also important to differentiate between hunger and thirst. Stomach hunger is your body's signal that you need to eat. Sometimes we feel physical hunger when we are actually in need of fluids and better hydration. Try drinking a glass of water and wait fifteen to thirty minutes to see if the hunger lessens or disappears.

This is an experiment that only you can perform. And like any good experiment, it should be repeated to confirm the results.

There is controversy among the experts about how much fluid an individual should drink each day. Several factors determine how much you need—body size, the amount of Calories consumed, the level of exertion or exercise, the weather, medication use, etc. The amount of fruits and vegetables consumed is also a factor, since these foods may contain eighty percent or more water.

Checking the color of your urine may be a quick way to evaluate your need for more liquid also. Look for a very pale color as a sign that you are adequately hydrated. But remember, shortly after you take a vitamin your urine may appear darker than usual, because of some of the compounds in the vitamin are being excreted in your urine. We have included a recommended amount of water in the *Recommended Daily Portion Guidelines* at the back of the book (see the Appendices). Use this as a guide to the minimum amount of liquids you should be consuming each day. You should consult your primary care provider for individual guidelines if you need to limit your fluids for medical reasons.

Hunger & Satisfaction Levels

Use this simple 1 to 5 scale to evaluate yourself:

5 Very Full
4 Slightly Full
3 Satisfied but Not Full
2 Mild to Moderate Hunger
1 Significant or Extreme Hunger

Write these numbers down in your log or food journal.

Listen with Body, Mind, and Spirit

Use your body, mind, and spirit to ask: What am I really experiencing— stomach hunger, eye hunger, heart hunger, or mind hunger?

Some helpful tips:

■ Practice eating until you are not quite satisfied. Wait 15 minutes and ask yourself again if you feel satisfied. This simple exercise can help to give you the confidence of eating slightly less than you're used to but knowing that in a few minutes you will be satisfied.

■ Eye hunger may occur when you see a tempting food—for example, when you pass a bakery, see a cookie jar, or walk by a buffet of beautiful food. It may happen after seeing a food-related commercial on TV. At first when you try to change your eating habits, it may make sense to change your eating environment. Avoid the sight of food temptations when you can.

■ Heart hunger or emotional hunger may happen when you are feeling stressed or tired and you eat to avoid strong emotions or to feel better. You may have become conditioned to use food as a sedative or a "pep pill." If you realize you aren't physically hungry, ask yourself, "What am I trying to feed?" Start to record your mood and thoughts in your journal.

Maggie Davis

Week 4 Daily Devotionals

Theme for the Week LISTENING

Verse to Memorize *But he who listens to me*
will dwell secure
and will be at ease,
without dread of evil.

—PROVERBS 1:33

Day 1 God Speaks in Many Ways

READ | Hebrews 1

In many and various ways God spoke of old to our fathers by the prophets. (v. 1)

We believe in a God who speaks! The opening verses of the Bible tell us that all creation came into being because "God *said*." And John picks up on this all-important theme in order to begin his own account of the life of Jesus: "In the beginning was the Word, and the Word was with God, and the Word was God" (John 1:1). We are familiar with the various promises throughout Scripture that assure us that God listens for the voice of his people, that he hears our prayers and is not deaf to the cries of our hearts. But complete fellowship with God means that we also listen to *his* words and that we learn to attune our ears to the sound of his voice.

This week's reflections focus on the various ways God speaks to us. "O that today you would hearken to his voice! Harden not your hearts," exhorts the psalmist (Psalm 95:7–8). Apparently, it is crucial for God's people to be able to discern the voice of their Lord. Otherwise, they may find themselves like wandering pilgrims, having in mind their distant goal, but knowing little if anything of God's guidance along the way. God has not left us to fend for ourselves in such a way.

From the beginning of creation God has spoken with his people. The Bible describes how God instructed Adam and Eve about living and enjoying Paradise. Even after they had sinned and guiltily hid from their Maker, they heard the voice of God calling to them in the garden (Genesis 3:9). The fruit of their disobedience to God's words, however, was the loss of the intimate, face-to-face conversation with God that they once knew. Since that time, people have had to learn to listen to God's Word through other means.

We know that, in the words of a widely popular Christian book, God "is there and he is not silent." The challenge is to become sensitive to his voice. It will not always come in tones that we readily expect or easily recognize.

God's call will often surprise us and may even cause us pain and dismay. But, the same voice that called out to the void and brought forth life still calls out to us . . . in many and various ways.

REFLECT | *During these past weeks, in what ways have you discovered God speaking to you? How can you become more sensitive to sound of his voice?*

Day 2   Listening to God's Prophet

READ | Exodus 20:1–26

You speak to us, and we will hear; but let not God speak to us, lest we die. (v. 19)

The nineteenth chapter of Exodus records that, in response to God's commands, the people of Israel promised Moses, "All that the LORD has spoken we will do" (19:8). Then, in order to confirm to the people that he indeed was speaking by Moses, God allowed them to hear the thunder of his mighty voice. But that experience was so terrifying that they wanted a less threatening way to hear from him. So, from that day forward they would never hear God's voice so directly again. God appointed the prophets to be the instruments of his voice—men and women who were so given to God, so yielded to his commands, that they could speak his word to the nation of Israel.

It was an awesome responsibility to be a prophet. The prophet was answerable to God for what he said, no matter how challenging his message. Naturally, some prophets found the task too difficult, so they would change or soften their words, or even make up a message that was more agreeable to the hearers. One of the marks of the true prophet was that he often warned the people about their sins, about the ways they were straying from God's ways or disobeying his voice. And he told them what would happen if they did not change. The false prophet was frequently more pleasant!

This gift of prophecy—of telling God's truth—did not stop with the coming of Jesus. According to the New Testament, there will be many who, by the inspiration of the Holy Spirit, will speak the divine message to God's people. When we hear someone deliver the word of the Lord, whether in a sermon, a teaching, or perhaps even in simple face-to-face conversation, are we attentive to it? Do we, like Israel, say, "All that the LORD has spoken we will do"? Or do we think to ourselves, "Who is this person who claims to be speaking for God?" There are still false prophets, of course, and we are not to be naïve. "Do not despise prophesying," writes Paul to the Thessalonians, "but test everything; hold fast what is good" (1 Thessalonians 5:20–21). The test of the true prophet is whether he or she exalts Jesus Christ and is faithful to the written Word of God. But we should be humble enough to listen for God's voice through the voices of his true servants, those whom he has called and anointed for that purpose. They have been given to the church to build us up in the faith and to help bring us to maturity in Christ.

REFLECT | *What are the hindrances you experience in hearing the word of the Lord through the voice of another person?*

Day 3   The Still, Small Voice

READ | 1 Kings 19:1–18
And after the fire a still small voice. (v. 12)

Only days before this experience, the prophet Elijah had won a tremendous spiritual victory at Mount Carmel over all the servants of Baal (1 Kings 18). Through their pleadings and gyrations the false prophets had worked in vain to prove the power of their god. Throughout that day, Elijah waited, even taunting them in their failure. Then, at the time of the evening sacrifice, he "repaired the altar of the LORD," which had fallen into disuse. The sacrifice was then prepared, and God answered his prayer by sending a fire from heaven that consumed the entire sacrifice, and the altar as well! The people were impressed, to say the least! "The LORD, he is God!" they cried over and over again. In the triumph of that moment, Elijah acted with boldness. He seized the 450 false prophets and had them slain on the spot, seeking to rid the nation of the false religion that was destroying them.

But Jezebel, the wicked queen and wife of King Ahab, sent Elijah an ominous message, swearing that she would do to him just what he had done to her prophets of Baal. Under the weight of that threat, Elijah's great faith abruptly collapsed into fear. He felt alone and vulnerable. He knew that, because of her influence over her husband, Jezebel had the power to make good on her threat. So Elijah fled from the capital city, a broken and fearful man, filled with self-pity and anger. In time, he came to a cave, and there he hid himself. There—precisely there, in the *midst* of turmoil—God met his anxious servant. First, God displayed his might in wind, earthquake, and fire—reminding Elijah that the reach of his arm is never too short to save his servants. Then came the real message, not in thundering noise and blazing sky, but in a still, small voice. The Almighty God, he who brought all creation into being at the sound of his voice, spoke to his servant in a whisper.

This story is important because we tend to look for God's entrance to be grand; we expect him to make his will known in the great and impressive displays of his miracles and his might. Our ears have grown deaf to the gentle voice within. God still speaks in our consciences, a little warning perhaps, a quiet reminder, a gentle direction of what he wants us to do. But unless we are attentive, we will hasten on. Looking for the big event, we may miss him altogether. In the small things of everyday, God is still speaking to those who will listen.

REFLECT | *Describe a time, perhaps recently, when you forgot what God had done in your life and you gave way to fear and anger. How can you become more keenly attentive to God's "still, small voice"?*

Day 4 The Voice of Jesus

READ | Mark 9:1–29

This is my beloved Son; listen to him. (v. 7)

Isn't it interesting that among the very few times we hear the voice of God in the New Testament—at Jesus' baptism (Mark 1:11); here, at Jesus' transfiguration on the mountain; and before his passion and death (John 12:28)—the only actual *command* God ever gives is this one: *listen?* Of all the things God could have told us to do with his Son, this is what he chooses: "listen to him." Why is that?

It is tempting to exempt ourselves from this directive. After all, the disciples were actually there, in the presence of God in the flesh. The voice of Jesus was as real to them as the voice of our best friend is to us. They spent three years in his company and under his instruction. The most common introductory phrase in the Gospels is "Jesus said. . . ." But hearing Jesus' voice is not the same as listening to his word. Remember, the disciples were often confused by Jesus' teachings. They frequently misunderstood his message and mistook his meaning. They may have heard the sound, but they often missed the sense.

It is not that we now understand everything Jesus said. Sometimes our minds and hearts are also confused. But we actually have the advantage of knowing, on this side of his death and resurrection, that Jesus is Lord (remember what we learned in Week 1), that his words are as alive and effective today as they ever were. *Today* we can listen to him, not in some vague, romantic way, not in some super-spiritual way, but as a living communication with a living Savior. "He speaks to me everywhere," wrote the hymnist. Perk up the ears of your heart today and listen for his voice. He is the Creator of all, and not only do the birds, the stars, the sun and moon "proclaim his praise," but also to the listening ear come intimations, thoughts, a sense of knowing—which we can learn to identify as his voice to us.

Inwardly digest his teachings and savor them as you read. They burned their way into the hearts of their hearers and later were "written down for our instruction" (1 Corinthians 10:11). Let them burn their way into your mind as a strong word of help and guidance. He speaks through them as well as through his living Spirit today. "He who has ears to hear, let him hear."

REFLECT | *Where have you had a "sense of knowing" that God is speaking to you this week? When and where is it easiest for you to hear God? Why?*

Day 5　Listening to Scripture

READ | 2 Timothy 3

All scripture is inspired by God and profitable for teaching, for reproof, for correction, and for training in righteousness, that the man of God may be complete, equipped for every good work. (vv. 16–17)

One of the chief instruments of God's voice to the world is the sacred Scripture of the Old and New Testaments. Through these written words, we "hear" the living word of God speaking to every generation. Everything necessary for our salvation is contained within their message.

Paul is giving some basic advice to young Timothy, his spiritual son in the faith. He knows that Timothy has been called upon to lead a group of Christians in the way of faith and obedience to God. Timothy himself had the privilege of associating closely with Paul. They, in turn, are in need of someone who has learned the faith and learned it well. So, Paul reminds Timothy that he has at his fingertips the tools he requires. Since childhood he has been acquainted with the Scriptures, and has seen them put into practice in the examples of his own mother and grandmother (1:5). Now that Timothy is "on his own," so to speak, Paul reminds him that it is these same words that will guard him against the false ways and tempting messages that he is encountering, even in the church of Christ.

The same is true for us today. Many erroneous and strange teachings are for sale in the Christian marketplace. Some of them sound very attractive, offering quick gratification and simple shortcuts to discipleship. Devoid of all "hard words," they promise us a cheap and easy way to holiness. Others play on guilt, or fear, or anxiety about the future, enslaving their adherents to legalistic methods or excessive practices. What is the defense against such error? The Holy Scriptures.

Read the Bible. Make yourself familiar with the "sounds" of its voice, for it is the voice of God himself. It is a treasure and storehouse of divine wisdom and truth, and through it God speaks to every condition of human life. "Thy word is a lamp to my feet and a light to my path," wrote the psalmist (119:105). With the gift of the Holy Spirit in our hearts, and undergirded by centuries of the Church's teaching, we can open the Scriptures confidently and expectantly so that we, too, may be "complete, equipped for every good work."

REFLECT | *In what ways this week has God directed your life through the Scriptures? When it comes to the Bible, how can you improve the quality of your listening to God's voice?*

Day 6   Listening to Circumstances

READ | Isaiah 30:8–33

And though the Lord give you the bread of adversity and the water of affliction, yet your Teacher will not hide himself anymore, but your eyes shall see your Teacher. And your ears shall hear a word behind you, saying, "This is the way, walk in it," when you turn to the right or when you turn to the left. (vv. 20–21)

God was speaking to his people through the circumstances of their lives. It was often the prophet's responsibility to make the connection between the things that God's people were experiencing and the things that God was saying to them. In times of blessing, the prophet pointed out the faithfulness of God and reminded them that they owed God all their thanks and praise. In times of trial, he discerned the chastening hand of God at work, and warned them to return to the ways of the Lord.

"'Woe to the rebellious children,' says the LORD, 'who carry out a plan but not mine,'" declares Isaiah at the beginning of this chapter. Israel, like us all, was insisting on having her own way, working out her own will, fulfilling her own desires. So, God visited Israel in a manner designed to get her attention—he came in the form of want and affliction.

The mystery of suffering cannot be explained by a simple equation, as if pain is always the product of sin (consider Job, for example). Nevertheless, we have the clear example of Israel, a people who, again and again, suffered the consequences of their rebellion against God's rule in their lives. Still, God kept watch, and, though he allowed circumstances of trouble and sorrow to afflict his people, his intention was always to do them good. "The LORD waits to be gracious to you," said his prophet (v. 18).

It is so with us. Insistence upon our own ways inevitably leads to confusion and distress. Most of us know from firsthand experience what that means. Through such circumstances, God is calling to us, compelling us to give up our own ways in favor of his. If our way is smooth and pleasant, let it be a reminder of how greatly we are loved, and let it spur us on to a more faithful love of our own. And, if our way is hard and we cannot see how it is going to work out for good, let us stop for a while, to listen, and to trust. "In returning and rest you shall be saved; in quietness and in trust shall be your strength" (v. 15).

Is my gloom, after all,
Shade of his hand, outstretched caressingly!
(*"Hound of Heaven," F. Thompson, 1859–1907*)

REFLECT | *Where, in the circumstances of your life, is God speaking to you? What is he saying?*

Day 7   Listening to Others

READ | Ephesians 4:15–32

Rather, speaking the truth in love, we are to grow up in every way into him who is the head, into Christ. (v. 15)

This week we have been reflecting on the various ways that God speaks to us, and on our need to attune the ears of our hearts to the many sounds of his voice. Today we consider one of those "sounds" that is the most difficult for us to hear: that of God speaking to us through the voice of another person.

"Let everyone speak the truth with his neighbor," writes the apostle Paul (v. 25). The Scottish poet Robert Burns wrote a little verse that says, "O wad [would] some Pow'r the giftie gie us, to see oursels as others see us!" As a matter of fact, Christians have been given that "giftie." If we are truthful with one another, we can see ourselves as others see us, and we can begin to get a better view of ourselves as God sees us.

Make no mistake; this is not always a pleasant revelation. We are reminded that what the prophet Jeremiah said about the human heart is true about our own hearts: "The heart is deceitful above all things, and desperately corrupt; who

can understand it?" (17:9). After a disagreement or a hurtful exchange of words, for example, my heart tells me that people don't understand me, that I really mean well, that I am right. But someone else listening in on the conversation sees things a different way and actually does me a favor by telling me so: "You know, what you said was really quite insensitive. Why are you so angry?" Such a word is hardly ever easy to hear, but if we will listen to those who speak such truth to us—even if we think they are not getting the whole picture (or that they may even be wrong themselves!)—a more truthful and complete view of ourselves will begin to be unveiled. That is the word of testimony of many people who have submitted themselves to the discipline of listening to others.

Our pride (even in its most timid form) is able to construct the most attractive but altogether false image of ourselves. The truth begins to tear away at that image and reveal the fragile threads that hold it together. This experience is painful, but it is valuable because both speaking and listening to what is *true* is the pathway to freedom—freedom from having always to sustain and protect a false image before the eyes of others, and freedom to have our souls re-created in the true image and likeness of Jesus. "A man who flatters his neighbor spreads a net for his feet" (Proverbs 29:5). Do we listen to flattery or to truth? Do we speak the truth in love, or do we spread nets for the feet of friends?

REFLECT | *What truthful thing about yourself is difficult for you to hear from another? What truthful thing should you be saying to a friend?*

Week 5 An Expression of Love

The Plan

EATING RIGHT

▪ "Break bread together" at dinner one time this week. Serve a loaf of whole grain, high fiber bread that everyone can tear off, instead of pre-sliced bread or rolls.

▪ Express love with food to your family this week, using one of Maggie's suggestions.

LIVING WELL

▪ Keep counting steps on your pedometer.

▪ Think of something special you want to do this week and do it! Maybe that will be a manicure or a pedicure. Or perhaps you would like to spend an hour visiting a bookstore or a library. Put something different into your routine this week to "live well."

LOVING GOD

▪ At a meal with friends or family this week, try something different when saying grace: put a written prayer of thanksgiving at each person's place, and take turns reading each prayer out loud.

An Expression of Love

WHAT IS OBEDIENCE? We all know what that means for training a child or a pet. But what does it mean for me? Is it even a relevant topic for today? Does obedience have a place in my daily life? Is it a little place or a big place? God gave some specific directions about the way we should live. But can we apply those directions to our eating habits?

The Ten Commandments give us definite "thou shalt" and "thou shalt not" instructions. But Jesus reinforced the Ten Commandments with even stronger words when he said that hating anyone is like murder, or looking at someone in lust is the same as adultery. How can I live an obedient life? The answer to this question has to come one day at a time.

What has God placed in front of me to train me in the way of obedience? Is it the "no parking" sign in front of the drug store that I ignore because I am just running in and out for two minutes? Is it the way I take my shoes off and leave them in the front hall instead of putting them away in my closet? Is it exceeding my food budget every week and hiding it from my husband? Is it driving over the speed limit?

What has God placed in front of me to train me in the way of obedience?

This week we'll be learning about obedience. From the earliest days of God's dealing with humanity, obedience has been a vital tool for a good life. Adam and Eve disobeyed God, and the result of their disobedience in this small thing—eating the forbidden fruit—continues to affect us all.

When God asks for obedience, he is not just referring to big issues. He is challenging us to be blessed by obedience in the smallest details of our lives. Where does God have the finger of conviction pressing on your heart? Are you ready to do something about it?

The 3D plan gives us many places to practice obedience, such as Maggie's suggestions about things we should do to live a more healthy life. What is God asking of you today?

Maybe it is time to realize that we are often more disobedient than obedient, and this may come as a surprise. After all, we are good people aren't we? We go to church, we pray, we don't smoke or swear or lie intentionally. Does your good-girl or good-boy list indicate who you really are in your heart? Or do you think of obedience as an outward action and not a choice of the heart? Let's go a little deeper this week to see how obedience is relevant to our everyday lives.

M. Cay Anderson use to say, "It's a golden diamond day when you find a sin hidden in your heart that you didn't know was there. It gives God a chance to wash it away." In week 5, we'll be looking at the blessing of obedience.

THE BLESSING OF OBEDIENCE begins with the knowledge that God loves us. We cannot understand obedience without first knowing how God loves us like a father—a good father who asks for our obedience so that we may grow into the people God wants us to be. In the *Your Whole Life* program, we redirect our lives, change our minds, and renew our relationships when we come to terms with the true, positive, holy way of obedience. Invite God to put his finger on those places where you have a disobedient heart and spirit. Then decide to listen carefully and take some action.

During this week, we will look at obedience as an expression of love. Any work or effort we begin requires obedience in order to reach the goal. Obediences of time, thought, and energy are required in order to achieve our goal. So, tell yourself, "I am going to be obedient to the disciplines I have undertaken." "I am going to be obedient to eat what I'm supposed to eat." "I am going to be obedient to treat my body, mind, and soul as prized possessions."

From now on, obedience and discipline should be positive words in your life!

Nothin' says lovin' like somethin' from the oven.

(Poppin' Fresh, the Pillsbury Doughboy)

Culturally and historically, the preparation and serving of food has been an expression of love, hospitality, nurturing, and caring. If food is love, how do you express your love for yourself, for your family and your friends through food? Is it more loving to serve a second vegetable at dinner or to bake a rich dessert and order a pizza? Positive eating habits and the love of healthy foods are a legacy that you can give to yourself, your family, and your friends. What better gift could we give, and what better expression of love could we offer, than those?

You may discover that you developed an unhealthy relationship with food or poor eating habits during childhood. **Even our health as adults is affected by the way we ate as children.** It is possible to modify our habits as adults. The greatest legacy for the children in your life may be the development of solid eating habits from an early age. If you're accustomed to treating your grandchildren or students in your class or the kids in your neighborhood with rich foods, it may seem awkward at first to express your love or appreciation by preparing and serving them healthy treats. (And I'm not saying that you should never serve or eat a sweet!)

The 3D plan not only means eating the right types and amounts of healthy foods, but it also encompasses the art of eating well by creating a designated eating area, setting the table, and establishing new routines for meals with family or when you're alone.

One reason that fast food is not as satisfying is that we usually eat it while on the run. If you're eating while driving, you may not actually see what you're eating. You can end up feeling as though you haven't eaten!

Most of us have routines that involve our health in the course of the day. Yours may include brushing and flossing once or twice a day, and taking medication or vitamins at specific times. Perhaps your routine includes a short walk or exercise. **As you begin to eat right and live well, you should examine your daily habits related to food, hospitality, and love, as well.**

Create New Ways of Eating Together

When I invite friends or family for dinner, I often urge everyone to "break bread" together rather than pre-slicing bread or serving tidy rolls. The sense of sharing this whole food adds another dimension of wholeness to a meal shared with those you love. And each person can tear off a portion that suits them.

I recall eating pizza in Naples and seeing that the Neapolitans don't pre-cut the pizza pie; instead, people tear apart their portions from the same pie. What a different experience from eating a precisely cut slice! This is an interesting concept that we could look at during these weeks. When we order a pizza, why not ask for it *not* to be sliced, and see if your choice would be smaller than usual? It is a temptation to eat a whole preportioned slice, when maybe we could tear off a small piece that would perfectly match our hunger.

When we look at things like this we become aware that someone else may indeed be telling us how much to eat, or giving us an excuse to eat more that we actually need. They are also inviting me to overeat. Everyone at my family table is not the same age, not the same gender, and not the same weight. **Why is every pizza slice the same size?** It is the same with an ice cream cone. The bigger the better for the same amount of money—that's why we look for the ice cream shop that scoops the most ice cream into a cone! Perhaps if enough of us demanded it we could insist on "kiddy cones" for adults. And instead of restaurants allowing "children's portions" only for those age six and under, we could begin to ask for a half-portion size. Some restaurants are doing this, and many others are charging a small additional fee for us to share an entrée.

I recently attended the funeral of a friend and nutritionist colleague. The numerous eulogies for her included the testimonials of wonderful meals that she had provided to family and friends who had eaten at her table, had shared her healthy foods, and had experienced fellowship with her through food. She embodied a healthy way of eating that became her way of expressing love through the medium of good food, served well. As a nutritionist, she had lived her life helping not only her patients and clients eat right but by demonstrating her love and affection by planning, preparing, and serving wonderful, nourishing meals. Eating right does not give immortality, but it can make your life richer in many ways.

Express Love with Food

Here are some helpful tips you can use to find your own healthy ways to express love with food:

■ Make your refrigerator into a take-out deli for healthy eating for yourself and your family.

■ Don't just buy fruit. Ripen it, peel it, and make it available as a fast food. Or buy it prepared at the supermarket salad bar. Go one step further and portion it into individual containers for quick snacks. Label it with the contents and the date it was made.

■ Make a batch of a vegetable soup each week that contains several vegetables and/or beans that can be microwaved for quick snacks or an appetizer while dinner is cooking.

■ Bake a batch of healthy oatmeal cookies including nuts and dried fruit, and make them small in size.

■ Set the table so that it is an attractive and appealing place to eat. Make your table look as though your meals are something special. And if your family meals have to be buffet-style because of school activities or different work schedules, use the table as an opportunity to say "I love you" to busy family members, with flowers, placemats, candles, and so on.

Maggie Davis

Week **5** Daily Devotionals

Theme for the Week   OBEDIENCE

Verse to Memorize   *He who has my commandments
and keeps them,
he it is who loves me;
and he who loves me will be loved
by my Father, and I will love him
and manifest myself to him.*
                                        —JOHN 14:21

Day 1   A Blessing and a Curse

READ | Deuteronomy 11:8–32

Behold, I set before you this day a blessing and a curse: the blessing if you obey the commandments of the LORD your God, which I command you this day, and the curse, if you do not obey the commandments of the LORD your God, but turn aside from the way which I command you this day, to go after other gods which you have not known. (vv. 26–28)

The Book of Deuteronomy (a word meaning "second law") is actually a repeat and summation of the instructions given by God to the children of Israel after their deliverance from Egypt and before their entrance into the Promised Land. One would expect, therefore, that this book would strike all the high points in God's relationship with his people. This can certainly be said of the words before us today—we must make a choice, and the result of that choice will be either blessing or curse. Obedience to the one, true God is the pathway to blessing; obedience to other "gods" is the pathway to ruin. Israel is being challenged to "choose life" (see Deuteronomy 30:19). Why is there such an emphasis on obedience?

God is not an unreasonable tyrant. He has not so constructed his world that he requires obedience for capricious reasons. The motivation behind his commands is his love:

everything that he asks of us is grounded in his love for us. We need always to look at the issue of obedience in this light. Consider children, for example. We all know that their natural desire is to do what pleases them, whatever will get them what they want, as soon as they want it. It is only with careful (sometimes painful) training that they learn that obeying mother and father brings more safety and satisfaction than getting away with whatever they want to do. Obedience brings blessing.

The sad story of the Old Testament, of course, is that of a people who, again and again, refused to be obedient to their God and suffered the consequences of their choices. God never abandoned them. He never ceased to look for ways to get their attention and return them to his ways. But what a lot of grief and suffering they could have been spared had they been obedient to his commands. Like them, we "children of God" are still learning God's ways. The same promise still holds: if we will be obedient to God, we will know his blessing. Start where you can! Keep at it! Don't give up! The blessing is worth it.

REFLECT | *What does the word "obey" mean to you? Where are you discovering the blessing of obedience in your life?*

Day 2   If You Love Me

READ | John 14:15–31
If you love me, you will keep my commandments. (v.15)

This is a strong and disturbing verse of Scripture. Jesus clearly states that obedience to his commandments is the expression and proof of our love. His statement is similar to said the one he made in the Sermon on the Mount, "Why do you call me 'Lord, Lord,' and not do what I tell you?" (Luke 6:46). Obedience is the unmistakable sign of allegiance to and love for Jesus Christ.

At this point in the Gospel of John, Jesus is facing the most severe trial imaginable—his passion and death. He is putting everything on the line for the sake of doing his Father's will, knowing that it will cost him his life. Is it any surprise that, in this very context, he would require the same of his disciples— and of us?

We need this sort of intense and direct word from time to time. Self-love is such a strong and sometimes hidden force that, unless something comes along to bring us up short, it can easily take over our hearts and crowd out our love for Jesus. Like the weeds in the parable of the sower, "the cares of the world, and the delight in riches, and the desire for other things, enter in and choke the word, and it proves unfruitful" (Mark 4:19).

"Yes, Lord; you know that I love you" is what Peter declared to Jesus when they met together on the beach after the Resurrection (John 21:15). This was not an answer spoken in haste, for Peter could still hear, with shame and sorrow, the words he had spoken when he had denied his Lord—"I do not know him"—even after promising that he would die for him if necessary. Here, in the forgiving presence of his Risen Lord, Peter could say, in spite of all he had done, and in spite of all he had not done, "Lord, you know everything; you know that I love you." From this point on, Peter's love for Jesus would be made evident by the obedience he rendered to his Master's command, "Feed my sheep."

Loving Jesus, and therefore, doing his will, is not something that we have the power to do in and of ourselves. That is his gift to us. With the apostle Paul, we can admit that without the help of the Holy Spirit within us, we are bound by the natural inclination to love ourselves above all else. The promise of the Gospel is that we can learn to have our lives directed by a new love, that we can actually become more interested in having God's will done than our own.

REFLECT | *How does your self-love express itself . . . specifically? How does the Holy Spirit help you to love God more than yourself?*

Day 3   You Will Abide in My Love

READ | John 15:1–11

If you keep my commandments, you will abide in my love, just as I have kept my Father's commandments and abide in his love. (v. 10)

Yesterday we considered how obedience is the decisive test of our love for Jesus. Obeying the will of God is the way we put hands and feet to our words, "Yes, Lord, you know that I love you." Today, the subject is turned around, and we are reminded of the

promise of what obedience will bring.

"You will abide in my love," says Jesus. What does this mean? At first glance, we may be tempted to think that Jesus is saying he will love us in exchange for our obedience.

For some reason—no doubt a combination of basic human nature together with experiences in our upbringing—we tend to think that "doing well" is the price of God's favor and approval. But this is clearly not the message of the Good News. God's love for us cannot be earned. It simply *is*.

For us to "abide" in Jesus' love is the same as his "abiding" in his Father's love. It means to be one in spirit with all that he is and all that he is doing. It means to live in the daily, moment-by-moment blessing of his grace and favor in our lives. In means that our lives are inseparably united with Jesus' life, just as Jesus' life is inseparably united with his Father.

Perhaps you have experienced a small taste of this with another human being. You loved that person, and as long as you and the other person were in unity of spirit, an atmosphere of freedom and trust endured between you. You wanted to please because you loved; and you were pleased because the other person loved you return. Each of your lives "abided" in the life of the other.

This is an inadequate but helpful picture of what Jesus is saying. Breaking his commandments brings about disjuncture, a fracturing of the relationship. Our own disobedience injures us, and therefore the relationship suffers, too. This does not mean that God ceases to love us; it does not even mean that we have ceased to love him. But it does mean that the intimacy of oneness is damaged, and therefore the blessing we knew in that oneness is cut off, waiting to be restored and renewed.

REFLECT | *Where in your own life do you know you have been willfully disobedient to God? What have been the results? What is it that you long for in your relationship with Jesus?*

Day 4   Whom Will You Serve?

READ | Romans 6:12–23

Do you not know that if you yield yourselves to any one as obedient slaves, you are slaves of the one whom you obey, either of sin, which leads to death, or of obedience, which leads to righteousness? (v. 16)

Here, in the sixth chapter of his letter to the Christians in Rome, Paul explains more about the intimate, almost organic, relationship between obedience and abiding in Christ. He draws upon a familiar image to illustrate his point—slavery. At its most basic, to be enslaved means to be bound to one's owner, obligated to choose only what accords with that master's will. Paul says that we fool ourselves if we think that we obtain freedom by doing whatever we please. "Wait until I'm eighteen," declares the angry young teenager. "Then I'll be free to do whatever I want." But the paradoxical truth is that, at just that moment when we exert our self-will with all our might, we are actually enslaving ourselves— yielding ourselves—to the forces of an altogether unreliable master, sin! We can choose our master, says Paul. But it will be one or the other—either sin or Christ. There is nothing in between.

This puts the matter quite plainly: we choose who is going to have dominion over us. At one time, we really had no choice. Paul says that, as the offspring of Adam and Eve, our fallen natures knew only one master—disobedience. But Jesus the Savior, God in the flesh, entered our world, took upon himself our human nature, lived a life of perfect obedience, and died with our sin upon his shoulders. Sin no longer reigns supreme over those who have been released from its clutches by the outstretched arms of Jesus. If the Key of David has unlocked our prison and set us free, why would we ever want to go back to captivity? Enslavement to sin leads ultimately to death. Enslavement to Jesus Christ leads to resurrection!

Someone may ask, "What kind of a choice is that—just a choice of masters?" To answer, we have only to look at where the other kind of slavery—slavery to sin—has taken us; or where it has taken others whom we know and love. Yielding ourselves to God does not mean that we lose the temptation to choose sin, nor does it mean that we have simply turned in one cruel master for another. In your service is perfect freedom, says an old prayer. To limit our choices to the will of God is actually to expand our world beyond all imagination. So, today, whom will you serve?

REFLECT | *It is in the nature of all of us to insist upon having our own way, but why are you insistent upon doing so? Describe for yourself the kind of freedom that you would like to experience in your life.*

Day 5   A Heavenly Vision

READ | Acts 26:1–32

Wherefore, O King Agrippa, I was not disobedient to the heavenly vision. (v. 19)

This week we are reflecting on the place of obedience in the Christian life. We know that, in this matter, all things are important, however small or large they may be. Learning to direct our wills in accordance with God's will is a lifelong endeavor, and every day we take the steps that lead us on that noble path, one at a time. Jesus said, "He who is faithful in a very little is faithful also in much" (Luke 16:10). This is why we need to try to see our disobediences from God's perspective.

Today's reading speaks of another dimension of obedience. Paul's obedience "to the heavenly vision" was an indispensable element in his *faithfulness* to Jesus Christ. Serving God was no longer simply a matter of doing right things and avoiding wrong things, as it had been in the days when he was a practicing Pharisee. A much larger vision now motivated Paul's obedience. God himself had called Paul into his service. He now had heaven before his spiritual eyes, and that bright vision compelled him to give all his heart and will— his entire life—to do the will of his Savior. When we think back to the fruit of that obedience (Paul was the first great Christian missionary!), it is impossible to overestimate the blessing he brought to the whole church of Christ. The example of his life, the words he spoke, and the letters he wrote make up some of the most valuable and helpful portions of the Holy Scriptures. The debt of gratitude owed to him by every generation of Christians is immeasurable.

"Where there is no vision," says the wise author of Proverbs, "the people perish" (29:18, KJV). Without this divine, long-range purpose toward which we can strive and move, life becomes mired in the concerns of the moment. Our spiritual muscles grow flaccid, our enthusiasm for the kingdom of God fades, and we lose our sense of direction. If you are taking the time to read these reflections, however, then you are probably aiming to live your life to the glory of God, and you, too, have a part in this "heavenly vision." There is a larger reason for you to be faithful than what you may presently think. In the eternal economy of God, your life and testimony matter to more people than you can imagine, or will ever know.

REFLECT | *List some ways you have sought to be obedient this week. What were the results? In what ways do you want your life to glorify God?*

Day 6　Be Subject to One Another

READ | Ephesians 5:1–33

Be subject to one another out of reverence for Christ. (v. 21)

Perhaps the hardest part of obedience is learning to submit our wills to the will of another. Put succinctly, none of us likes to be told what to do! We fear that to submit ourselves to another person will lead to the loss of our freedom, the smothering of our own desires and, ultimately, to the annihilation of our own personalities. These fears may be unfounded and even unreasonable, but they are real nonetheless, and they are very difficult to subdue. And they prevent us from availing ourselves of one of the greatest gifts God has given to his people—his own guidance through the lives of one another.

This is because we think that our security and well-being depend upon strength and power. But remember what Jesus said when Pilate asked him if he did not realize that Pilate had the power to put him to death: "You would have no power over me unless it had been given you from above" (John 19:11). The only power that matters is God's. And, if each of us is in God's hands, then it is not only safe but it is beneficial to "be subject to one another out of reverence for Christ." In the kingdom of God, strength is not the determining factor as to whose way prevails. The strong are to serve the weak, and those who are weak may actually be the strongest of all. Therefore, Paul instructs wives to be subject to their husbands "as to the Lord," and husbands to lay down their lives (including their own wills) as Christ laid down his life for the Church. No one, then, is to be lording it over anyone else. Rather, there is to be a mutual preference for one another. Jesus said, "The kings of the Gentiles exercise lordship over them; and those in authority over them are called benefactors. But not so with you; rather let the greatest among you become as the youngest, and the leader as one who serves" (Luke 22:25–26).

If we are subjecting ourselves to one another out of reverence for Christ, this means that we are hearing what Jesus has to say to us through another person. If we become suspicious enough of our own willful tendencies, we will not be so afraid to consider the thoughts of another, nor so resistant to put down our own will in order to do what someone else suggests. This is not an easy assignment, and, to be sure, it requires both trust and love—trust in God and love for one another. "Walk in love, as Christ loved us," wrote Paul (v. 2). Speaking of strength and power, being subject to one another out of reverence for Christ is one of strongest expressions we have of love for our "neighbor," and one of the most powerful testimonies we can offer to the world of our love for God.

REFLECT | *What do you fear most about "subjecting" yourself to others? What do you have to gain by overcoming that fear?*

Day 7   Faith Without Works

READ | James 2:8–26

So faith by itself, if it has no works, is dead. (v. 17)

Through this past week we have considered many different aspects of what it means to be obedient to God: obedience as the path to blessing, as an expression of our love for Christ, and as the way to God's abiding presence; obedience as the inescapable choice about whom we will serve, together with the consequences of that choice; obedience as faithfulness to a vision that is larger than a list of dos and don'ts. We have even thought about the problem of subjecting ourselves to others, and finding God's will in what another person might tell us to do. Today we touch upon one final aspect.

The letter of James was written to a group of Christians who insisted that faith alone was all they needed and who disregarded the necessity of active obedience to the truth. The author is greatly concerned that they (we) see the deception of such thinking. Where faith is alive, he says, works (read "obedience") will follow. If there are no works—no loving deeds, no sacrificial offerings, no helpful services—this can only be because there is no genuine faith. Doing good things is not the way we earn our way into God's favor. However, once we come to know the love of God and to believe that he has a will for our lives, then works become the mandatory demonstration of faith, the clearest evidence we can give that God has entered our lives.

This brings us back to the basic struggle we all face as Christians. It is the struggle between the disobedient "self-centered"—with all its stubborn and devious methods for getting its own will—and the obedient "self-less" with its disarming simplicity and faithful compliance to God's will. All of us face this struggle every day and, as we strive to subdue the former and strengthen the latter, we find that we understand better the nature of the struggle going on within us.

Do not be lax, therefore, in your efforts to put your faith into practice.

Thank God for a living faith that can produce living works as its fruit! In this way we are truly following in the obedient footsteps of our Lord and Savior, Jesus Christ.

REFLECT | *Describe any struggle that might have gone on within you this week between the "self-centered" and the "self-less" in you. In what ways did you find obedience to God to be a blessing this week?*

THOUGHT   66 Change your thoughts and you change your world. 99

(Norman Vincent Peale, 1898–1993)

Week 6 The Challenge of Change

The Plan

EATING RIGHT

- Examine your journal for clues of rebellion regarding food. How can you constructively deal with resentment, rather than with food?

- Try one new, healthy food this week—an unusual fruit that is in season, or a new way of cooking an ordinary vegetable.

- On your next trip to the grocery store, try shopping only in the outside aisles where most of the whole foods are found.

LIVING WELL

- Do you have a goal for steps each day? Why not set a daily realistic goal and endeavor to make it? Try walking somewhere new, such as the public gardens, the beach, or a bike trail.

- Take an extra five minutes to get yourself ready in the morning. Investing a little extra time in your personal appearance will build self-respect and help you start the day on the right foot.

LOVING GOD

- Brother Lawrence, in his classic book *The Practice of the Presence of God*, finds a relationship with God in the most ordinary details of life. This week, as you go about your everyday routine, look for God in the details. Doing the laundry, waiting in line at the grocery store, or chopping carrots can all become occasions for rehearsing your Scripture memory verse and connecting with God.

THOUGHT **"** A man's palate can,
in time, become accustomed to anything. **"**

(Napoleon Bonaparte, 1769–1821)

The Challenge of Change

WEEK 6 MAY BE THE TIME WHEN the 3D plan begins to feel really *difficult*! The early victories and fresh feelings of change wear off, and it is time to commit to the challenge to change and persevere as God wants you to.

This week could be a difficult time for you. Our own natures get in the way at times like this: if we have not lost the weight we wanted to lose, if we feel discouraged, if we are finding it hard to keep trying—this is the point where we want to quit! I've been there myself. That may be how you are feeling this week.

> This week could be a difficult time for you.

However, don't give up. Millions of women and men before you have gotten to the sixth week and have wanted to give up. Somehow, they have persevered, and they were enormously glad that they did so! This is a daily journey. There are going to be some downs. There are going to be weeks when you just don't feel like going to a meeting, or exercising, or sticking to food disciplines.

It's okay to feel that way and to go through those times. In diet-talk, this week may be a plateau for you. There are also spiritual plateaus and emotional plateaus. You may be at one. If you are, grab hold, pray, and let's go on! Share with someone, perhaps someone in your group, that you are feeling discouraged. Tell at least one other person, and it will release the power of defeat.

Twenty years ago, I visited a health awareness hospital in Napa Valley, California. Their entire program centered on health and wholeness. I remember clearly the talk on habit-changing. It takes twenty-one days to change a habit, they told me. This was a new insight for me. That means three weeks without slipping back. This is harder than it sounds.

The other thing I learned was that we form habits in order to save the brain's energy. How many times have you picked up a candy or put something in your mouth that you didn't mean to do? It just happened. That was a habit for me at work. That was news to me twenty years ago, but it helped me understand the hard work it takes to change habits.

The illustration the doctor gave was the building of a new highway. Workers have to clear land, cut down trees, dig up stumps, and truck in lots of new materials. Many roads are created through solid rock or deep woods. To create new habit patterns one needs to work as hard to construct a new road in the brain as it takes construction workers to build a new highway. We work, work, and work, and many times it just doesn't look like there will ever be a new highway. Then one day you realize you are on a new road.

Your new roadway is under construction; don't give up. Six more weeks will reinforce the new choices you have been making.

Don't Turn Back Now!

As we approach the halfway point in our twelve-week program you may be wondering if all this work is really worth it. You may even find yourself formulating excuses for not continuing to change your life. Some of the little devils and or big demons that may have sabotaged you in the past may be trying to come back into your thoughts now. "It's too expensive to eat right," my clients sometimes complain. Or, "You have to be in good shape to exercise." And I often hear, "I have too many responsibilities to focus on my own needs." These are all instances of self-talk that keep you from eating right. Maybe it's time to give yourself another permission slip!

After five weeks of changes in diet and exercise you may complain, "But I'm only losing a pound a week, and I want to lose 50 pounds!" Although the results of your changes may not be as dramatic as you'd like, if you are able to sustain your new habits and make additional changes along the way, you may be able to lose 50 pounds in one year or so, and you will be more likely to keep the weight off permanently than if you lose 20 pounds the first month only to "burn out" on an overly restrictive weight-loss diet.

Behavior modification research shows that conditioning and establishing a new habit generally takes 21 days to become a part of your usual routine. If you break the habit at day 13, you will need to start over and continue for another 21 days to firmly establish the habit. For this reason it may be easier for you to pick one or two things to work on rather than tackle too many food and exercise changes all at once. In reality, it may take a full three months to really own a new habit if you realize that you may try, relapse, and need to try again. If your mind, body, or spirit is rebelling at this point, it may be because you are making too many changes at once and not "owning" any one change completely. You may need to revise your goals or revisit previous chapters.

Change Is Good

Now may be a time to look at the variety of foods you are eating. Are you bored with your meals? Are you

Tips for Men

Your body is made up of anywhere from fifty to seventy-five percent water, making water the largest compound by far. You get water primarily from consuming liquids and from the food you eat. Since vegetables and fruits are mostly water, they may contribute significantly to your overall fluid intake. **Try to pay attention to your thirst (especially when the temperature is high or you are engaging in physical exercise or sports) and respond by drinking water.** In general, men need about three quarts of liquid per day from water and beverages. However, be conscious of the potential Calories you may consume if you drink juices, sodas, alcoholic beverages, sweetened tea, or sports drinks. Liquid Calories may not give you the same satisfaction as chewing the same number of Calories. In addition, high glycemic sugared beverages and alcoholic beverages can even make you hungrier.

tired of eating similar meals each day even though you consider them safe choices? If you are feeling that you can't eat like this forever, you may need more variety each day.

One way to evaluate your meals is to look at the color on your plate. Is everything white or beige or green? Are you eating peas every day because you don't like other vegetables? (Men, in particular, may identify with this.) Are you shopping for the same fruits even when they are out of season?

Keeping variety in your meals and snacks is not only nutritionally sound, but also keeps your meals interesting and satisfying.

Consider the way that change happens. Change is a dynamic process that keeps you moving forward, even helping you to get back on the road if you derail at times. Don't become discouraged by your relapses; they are not failures unless you allow them to become permanent by not setting yourself back on the right course once again.

The Change Cycle

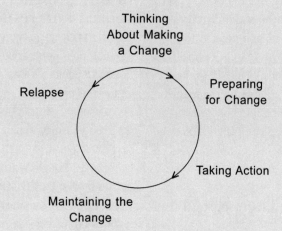

Thinking About Making a Change

Relapse

Preparing for Change

Taking Action

Maintaining the Change

Maggie Davis

Week 6 Daily Devotionals

Theme for the Week REBELLION

Verse to Memorize *Behold, to obey is better*
than sacrifice, and to hearken
than the fat of rams.
For rebellion is
as the sin of witchcraft,
and stubbornness is as
iniquity and idolatry.
—1 SAMUEL 15:22B–23 (KJV)

Day 1 Mutiny Amidst the Bounty

READ | Genesis 2:15–17; 3:1–24

[God] said . . . "Have you eaten of the tree of which I commanded you not to eat?"
(3:11)

Last week we focused on the theme of "obedience"—one of the primary ways in which we put our faith to work, both a result and a proof of our love for God and for one another. This week, we turn over the coin to look at the other side, and it is a dark side. *Rebellion* is not a pleasant word, much less a pleasant idea. And it is not a word we would readily use to describe our state of mind and heart before God. Nevertheless, it is the most "natural" part of our condition as human beings. To rebel against God and his ways is simply an inherent piece of human nature. Recall the universally understood words of the apostle Paul: "For I do not do the good I want, but the evil I do not want is what I do" (Romans 7:19).

The history of our beginnings is recorded in the book of Genesis (*genesis* means "origin") in the form of a series of stories. These are the stories of God's great love and power in creation, of the making of man and woman, and the abundant blessings they enjoyed in Paradise. Eventually, they are the stories of human pride and jealousy, of fear and deception, even of hatred and murder. Nevertheless, in between the bounty and the barrenness, there occurs a singular, seemingly insignificant event that sets all humanity on its course to ruin. This is why the story of Adam and Eve's rebellion—doing that which God had commanded them not to do— is called "The Fall."

This week, we will be reflecting on the reality of rebellion in the human race, and of our own specific part in it. Rebellion brings penalty according to God's law, not because he is capricious, but precisely because he cares so very much. As Lord of the universe, he set humanity upon a course of blessing. Our first parents turned that course into a trail of curses. "The LORD is in the right," said the prophet Jeremiah; the rebel is in the wrong (Lamentations 1:18). Humanity cannot excuse its mutiny against God's government, and we cannot excuse our own rebellion against what we know God requires of us. What is sown is reaped, and the effects can be heartbreaking, as we know from Genesis and, perhaps, as we know from our own experience.

Therefore, it should neither surprise nor dismay us when we see the results of our rebellion displayed in our life situations, in our personal lives, in our relationships, even in our children (remember the sons of Adam and Eve). Nevertheless, we can face directly this "dark side" of the coin because we know that the story of God's dealings with humanity does not end with the Book of "Origins." A new beginning commenced with the coming of Jesus Christ. "Thanks be to God"! (Romans 7:25).

REFLECT | *What experiences have you had, or do you now have, that you can see are the results of your rebellion against God's ways? Adam and Eve offered excuses for their rebellion—what excuse(s) do you make?*

Day 2   A Stubborn Generation

READ | Psalm 78:1–20

And that they should not be like their fathers, a stubborn and rebellious generation, a generation whose heart was not steadfast, whose spirit was not faithful to God. (v. 8)

The psalmist relates a parable, a "dark saying from of old," that he had heard from "our fathers" (vs. 1–3). It is both the sad story of Israel's rebellion and the glorious story of God's faithfulness. The songwriter presents a kind of *Reader's Digest* condensed version of Israel's history, citing the wonderful deliverances of God and the constant tendency of the people to turn away from him. As we read this psalm, however, we are aware that it is more than the story of an ancient people and their God. It is also the story of our own rebellion and of God's judgments and mercies in our lives. We know from our reading yesterday that, just as God's faithful ways are consistent, so also—at least on this side of heaven—are the stubborn ways of human nature.

In his letter to the Romans, the apostle Paul discusses the Israelites' failure to keep God's law; in fact, he describes their inability to do so. With the fall of Adam and Eve, he argues, all generations are consigned to their own rebellious ways and to the disastrous consequences of those ways. He concludes, therefore, that the law declares us all equally guilty before God—Jew and Gentile alike—and, therefore, all are equally in need of God's mercy and forgiveness. (It can be a bit daunting, but try reading straight through Romans 5–8 sometime.)

So, how is it that God deals with the rebellion of his people? The psalmist writes: "He established a testimony in Jacob, and appointed a law in Israel" (v. 5). This was God's first move, to set up the evidence of his merciful deliverance (the "testimony") and to make clear what he required of those whom he chose to be his own people. Here we see the compassion of God, and his infinite patience with the people he has chosen and loved. The marvels he wrought in Egypt, the manna he provided in the wilderness, and the water he sent forth from the rock—these all should have been ample testimony of his care. Still, even in the face of such unmistakable wonders, the people "sinned still more against him" (v. 17).

What about the testimony, the witness of God's mercy in *our* lives? How long do we remember the good things that God has done for us? And when we forget them, how long does it take us to reassert our stubborn wills and to rebel against what we know to be God's "law" for our lives? That is the question. For he has established a testimony, a record of loving deeds for us as surely as he did for Israel of old.

REFLECT | *What "testimony" has God established in your own life that declares his love and faithfulness to you? In what specific ways are you "stubborn" against God's will for your life?*

THOUGHT 66 I know, O Lord, and do with all humility acknowledge myself as an object altogether unworthy of thy love; but sure I am, thou art an object altogether worthy of mine. Do thou then impart to me some of that excellence, and that shall supply my own lack of worth. Help me to cease from sin according to thy will, that I may be capable of doing thee service according to my duty. 99

(St. Augustine, 354–430)

Day 3   Relentless Rebellion

READ | Psalm 78:32–72

Yet they tested and rebelled against the Most High God, and did not observe his testimonies, but turned away and acted treacherously like their fathers.
(vv. 56–57a)

The latter half of Psalm 78 catalogues the folly of continued rebellion in the face of God's dealings with his people. His "destroying visitations" to them succeeded in producing only their temporary return to God. "When he slew them, they sought for him; they repented and sought God earnestly" (v. 34). However, their repentance was short-lived, and soon the pull of the old ways was stronger than their fear of God's judgments. Repeatedly they "rebelled against him in the wilderness and grieved him in the desert" (v. 40).

Does this sound at all familiar? How steadfast are we in following God's ways, regardless of our circumstances? Like the pilgrim people of Israel, do we return and earnestly seek the Lord in times of affliction, only to forget his ways after he has answered and life returns to "normal"? When he meets us in our weakness, we find his mercy flowing freely, but then, once we are back on our feet, we find that our self-will and old habits pull us strongly against what we know to be the will of God.

The depth and resilience of our rebellious nature is something that we must confront, for it will always find a way to thwart even our best intentions to follow God. Rebellion's relentless force is one of the reasons it is important to allow others to have some authority in our lives, to give them permission to tell us what to do in one or more areas. Without such assistance, we can easily fool ourselves into thinking that we are doing everything the Lord wants us to do, when in reality we are simply having our own way.

The dominion of Israel was finally lost, rejected by God because of her rebellion. Only the lowly tribe of Judah remained to carry on the testimony of God. In the end, God would have his way even if his people would not. The sad account made by the writer of Psalm 78 stands as a permanent warning to us of the effect of persistent rebellion against a Holy God. The problem of rebellion is a serious matter in the kingdom of God. Tomorrow we will discuss just how dark it is seen by the eyes of heaven.

REFLECT | *Determined self-will and recurring habits often rob us of spiritual gains. How does the strength of your own rebellion exhibit itself? How can you better cooperate with God in your daily life so that you can choose God's will?*

Day 4   Rebellion: As Dark as All That?

READ | 1 Samuel 15

For rebellion is as the sin of divination, and stubbornness is as iniquity and idolatry. (v. 23a)

The story of Saul's rebellion is essentially the story of human pride and arrogance. Simply stated, Saul put his own judgment ahead of God's clear command. After doing battle in the name of God, he defied the will of God, and determined that his own point of view was actually better than heaven's. Saul reasoned that, since Agag was king, he should not be destroyed along with other Amalekites. Furthermore, killing perfectly good sheep, oxen, fatlings, and lambs— as he had been instructed to do (v. 3)—did not make sense to him. He disobeyed God's specific command without blinking an eye. In his self-delusion, he even had the audacity to declare before Samuel, "I have performed the commandment of the LORD" (v. 13).

"What then is this bleating of the sheep in my ears, and the lowing of the oxen which I hear?" asked Samuel. The evidence against Saul was indisputable, no matter how many self-defensive rationalizations he offered. Living flesh and blood testified against him. So he tried a blatant lie in order to justify his disobedience, to make his bad choices look good: "My plan was to make a special sacrifice to the LORD." Hogwash! Samuel saw right through Saul's deceptions and pressed him further: "Why then did you not obey the voice of the LORD?" What mattered to the prophet more

than to the king was obedience to the clear command of the Lord.

At this point, Saul did a very interesting thing (not at all unlike what we do when we are confronted with our wrong). He said, "I *have* obeyed. . . . I *have* gone on the mission. . . . I *have* brought Agag. . . . I *have* utterly destroyed. . . . *But the people . . .*" (v. 20–21). Does this sound familiar? In order to excuse his own disobedience, he put the blame on "the people." (Can you hear the echo of Adam's voice: "the woman whom thou gavest"?)

There is an all-important lesson for us in this passage. Rebellion against the will of God is rooted in one proud idea that has been with us since the Garden of Eden: "I know best." And, to our further detriment, upholding this idea inevitably leads to all kinds of reasoning, rationalization, and excuse-making. By such mental gymnastics, we may actually convince ourselves (and maybe even a few others) that we are obeying God. But make no mistake. If we truly want God's will for our lives, there has to be a reckoning time. Our rebellion must be addressed. Better that we confront it soon, before it has time to do its destructive work in us and in others around us. Equating it with witchcraft and sorcery is intended to show us its true darkness, so that we may turn from it with abhorrence.

REFLECT | *In what ways have you rationalized your behavior or your decisions? When was the last time you blamed someone else for your own actions or attitudes?*

Day 5   Do Not Harden Your Hearts

READ | Hebrews 3

But exhort one another every day, as long as it is called "today," that none of you may be hardened by the deceitfulness of sin. (v. 13)

Someone has said with regard to these verses: "Tomorrow is the day when idle men and fools repent. Tomorrow is Satan's today; he cares not what resolutions you form, if only you fix them for tomorrow." Whenever God leads us to a step of forward progress in our life of personal discipline and obedience, the tempter whispers, "You don't have to do that today. This one time won't matter that much. It can wait." Whenever we are tempted to ignore or to outright disobey one of the disciplines we know that God is requiring of us, the same soft murmur comes into our minds. You may be hearing it a lot these days.

Consistently giving in to such temptation is what leads to being hardened by "the deceitfulness of sin," as the writer to the Hebrews puts it. The old pattern of disobedience is continued. It becomes fixed as a kind of "conditioned response" to a given situation. For example, something happens that makes us feel sorry for ourselves, or we get angry or resentful, we are disappointed by people or circumstances, or our feelings are hurt by the thoughtlessness of a loved one. In such a case, look out! These are prime opportunities for the tempter to come and whisper, "Take a break. You can resume your discipline tomorrow. Today, you need to take care of yourself. Obviously no one else is going to." The problem, of course, is that "tomorrow" turns into next week, which turns into next year . . . which can turn into never.

In order to strengthen our wills to do God's will, it is essential that we see this part of human nature, and learn to guard ourselves against it. "Exhort one another every day," says the writer. The truthful voice of others to you—and your own voice offered for the sake of another—can help to drown out the quiet lies of temptation. And even when those attractive whispers do get through, a cry for help to family or friends can bring the help we need to stay the course. We need not fight rebellion on our own.

Take heart, but also take warning from what the writer to the Hebrews is saying. The heart that is hardened through the deceitfulness of sin only leads us to situations that are more painful later on. Since God is working with us to bring us more fully into conformity with his will, we must expect that he will keep on working, in many and various ways, to soften our hearts and to clarify our vision, so that we will not be fooled by rebellion's sneaky ways.

REFLECT | *What temptations do you encounter when you feel sorry for yourself, when you are angry, or when you are resentful? Describe a time when you asked, or someone asked you, for help to overcome such temptation.*

Day 6   Remember Korah

READ | Numbers 16
Therefore it is against the LORD that you and all your company have gathered together; what is Aaron that you murmur against him? (v. 11)

Korah and his followers stand as extreme examples of unbridled rebellion, in both attitude and action. And the terrible consequence of their rebellion presents a graphic warning to the people of

Israel and to all who would stubbornly defy the holy authority of God. Their story depicts just how destructive is rebellion's inevitable outcome. At the hand of Korah and his faction, a conspiracy is hatched, challenging the leadership of Moses and Aaron. Here are some thoughts for our meditation:

First, their rebellion was rooted in their jealousy. When we find ourselves inwardly resisting or resenting those in places of leadership, we should be suspicious of our own motivation. Jealousy is an insidious sin that quickly grows, feeding on small dissatisfactions, consuming all good will, and, at times, resulting in major crises. This sin does more harm to the harmony of Christian fellowship than any other. It is not insignificant that the first act of sin recorded after the Fall—Cain's murder of Abel—was prompted by jealousy (see Genesis 4:1–8).

Second, Korah's rebellion was sustained, even strengthened, by murmuring and backbiting. The dictionary defines backbiting as "saying mean and spiteful things about a person who is absent." Jealousy uses backbiting in order to do its destructive work. In the end, its desire is to put down the other for the sake of raising up oneself. Rebellion could not become conspiracy without it.

Third, those who were engaged in the rebellion were the only ones who were ultimately harmed. God has pledged himself to protect and defend his work. What he has begun he promises to complete, and the Bible makes it clear that the arm of flesh is too weak to thwart his designs. Therefore, if we place ourselves, even unwittingly, against what God is doing, we endanger our very own interests, for our good is central to his plan. In every gathering of faithful Christians— every church, congregation, fellowship, or small group it is important to guard ourselves against jealousy and its proud offspring, rebellion. Every discipline we undertake for the sake of doing God's will carries with it the temptation to resist and rebel. So, in light of what we see in Korah and his followers, let us pray fervently and behave wisely, that we may be instruments for accomplishing God's plan and not obstacles to it.

REFLECT | *Whose influence and direction in your life do you have the most difficulty following? Why? Where are you aware that jealousy is clouding your perception of God's will?*

Day 7   The Sour Fruit of Rebellion

READ | Romans 1:18–32

And since they did not see fit to acknowledge God, God gave them up to a base mind and to improper conduct. (v. 28)

Even knowing the redemptive grace of God as we do, we must admit that the topic of rebellion is neither pleasant nor easy to face directly. As we have seen this week, rebellion certainly figures prominently in the Bible's account of human sin. Still, it seems to be of the very nature of rebellion to downplay itself before our eyes and to fool us into thinking that our willful ways cannot possibly be as bad as all that. So, before moving on to other things, we must confront one more aspect of rebellion's ugliness.

This section of Paul's letter to the Romans has been aptly referred to as the darkest description of human nature in the Bible. The apostle's aim is to lay out the stark and shocking results of unchecked rebellion. He wants his readers to be disgusted by the actions of men and women who, by rebelling against God's law, have abandoned themselves to their basest cravings. This is what it means to be a rebel apart from the grace of God.

We are confronted here with an aspect of God's holiness that largely remains shrouded in mystery for us—his wrath. Because our own anger is so infected by impure motives and self-centered affections, it is difficult for us to comprehend an anger that is wedded to pure love. God's anger is directed against sin—in other words, against all that would do harm to the souls of his beloved. Paul tells us that, whether they know it or not, everyone's conscience can recognize God's holiness. However, by continually rebelling against God, the conscience eventually becomes so seared and deadened that it can no longer respond to

God's wrath. "Willful resistance to light," says David Brown, "has a retributive tendency to blind the moral perceptions and weaken the capacity to apprehend and approve of truth and goodness; and thus is the soul prepared to surrender itself, to an indefinite extent, to error and sin."

The key phrase is "willful resistance to light." We are not responsible for what we have not been taught, but we certainly stand accountable for what we know to be true. "The times of ignorance God overlooked," says Acts 17:30, "but now he commands all men everywhere to repent." In other words, we are morally and spiritually responsible for the light we are given. This is true of both the welcome light that warms our souls as well as the often unwelcome light that convicts our hearts. (More about this next week.) Instead of struggling against the light, we should struggle against ourselves. The sour fruit of rebellion, when God gives a person up to the lusts of the heart, is both frightening and deadly. Let it compel us to put down our own resistance and to give ourselves up to the will of God, by whatever means he makes it known to us.

REFLECT | *Think about those specific places in your life where you are rebellious. Have you discovered any habit patterns that encourage your rebellion? What are they? What helps you most to embrace the will of God?*

The Plan

EATING RIGHT

- Make a note in your journal of all the places where you eat meals or snacks.

- Plant some herbs or vegetables in a garden or a flower pot, or buy a small pot of herbs in the grocery store.

- Using the Whole Food Continuum on page 156, substitute one or two whole foods in place of foods that are highly refined or more processed.

LIVING WELL

- "Living Well" is extremely important, but it is different and personal to each individual. Write in your journal this week what "living well" would involve for you. Would it be listening to music? Visiting family or friends? Working in your garden? Watching a fun TV show? Going to the movies? Reading a book?

- *Do* something different this week that says, "This is 'living well.'"

- Keep walking!

LOVING GOD

- This week, in addition to your devotional readings and Scripture verse memorization, try opening up to someone in a new way. Sharing your feelings, struggles, hopes, and prayers with someone else opens the door to a deeper relationship, and it invites honesty in return.

Finding the Balance

MANY YEARS AGO THERE WAS A POPULAR PHILOSOPHY that said, "I'm okay, you're okay." Most of us loved it, didn't we? This slogan communicated that we shouldn't interrupt each other's lives with words that would throw us off balance; we should accept each other just as we are.

Most of us have indeed lived that way with family and friends and even at church. "Hi, how are you?" we hear regularly in our day. "Just great, how are you?" we answer. And we both go on our separate ways. Did the person really want to know how I was? And did I really want to tell her? I am not saying that everyone who asks you this question needs to listen to your troubles or that you have to share your struggles with anyone who asks. But we should consider seriously what it means to be open and honest. As we address this subject, my challenge to you is to use your group of friends to go a step deeper in your life.

We are off balance when we pretend that everything is fine when it isn't. I have faith that we can help each other when we begin to be truly honest. Honesty can be simply admitting that you fell off your "eating right" regime, or that you are fearful and upset and not sure you can make all these changes in your life. It could even be a prayer request that you can't talk about but for which you deeply want the prayers of your friends. Only you know what you can speak openly about with others and what must remain private. But most of us need to take steps to be more open and honest about what we can share—and then we should expect God to have words of encouragement and words of faith from our friends.

> We are off balance when we pretend that everything is fine when it isn't.

In my job at a Christian publishing house, I work with a lot of younger women. Sometimes I arrive at work in turmoil about something, and my work is affected. I might want to wait until I get home and call an older friend to talk over what is upsetting me, but I find that if I trust God and tell my co-workers what is on my heart, God will speak to me through them. Waiting until I can find the "right" friend to talk with will waste a lot of God's time. It has never failed that one of these young women has just the words I need to hear at that moment.

Openness and honesty bring wholeness. I encourage you to try it today.

Personalize Your Strategies

During the last six weeks you may have devoted a great deal of time and attention to planning, purchasing, and preparing healthy meals. You have started to become more aware of how you eat and the factors involved in your eating behaviors. But by now real life has re-entered your quest to eat right. You may have stopped gaining weight and perhaps lost some weight, or you may have reached a plateau. Now is the time to evaluate if the changes you are making are becoming part of your whole life.

Healthy eating means that you eat when you are hungry and that you are satisfied when you are finished. It also means that you give some thought to what you are going to eat and how much. You may have found that you are able to listen to your body's signals of hunger and fullness and maintain a healthy diet in response. Others find that their appetites are not reliable guides to how much to eat due to the effect of medication, a medical condition, or emotions. **If you feel that you fit into this latter category, you may need to consult with a professional to pinpoint the exact cause and possible additional treatment.**

Occasionally having a splurge or breaking from your usual routine does not need to amount to a relapse. It simply means that you will quickly need to get back on track and not let a big splurge or even a slightly larger portion become a new routine. **Continuing to evaluate your portion sizes is your insurance for keeping on track.** You must also be aware that as you lose weight your body will need fewer Calories, since you are not working as hard to carry around the weight that you have lost. Therefore, the portions that you consumed while you were first losing weight may now need to be re-evaluated. You may need to make your existing portions just slightly smaller. By making changes slowly, you will avoid giving your body the signal that it is starving. You are also less likely to feel deprived if you adapt to small changes gradually.

Nutrition for You, Your Family, and Beyond

Finding your own balance may also involve integrating the way you eat with that of your family, friends, and co-workers. How does the rest of your family eat, and how do your needs fit in? Is there anyone in your family or household who doesn't need to make healthier food choices? Making changes gradually for you and those who you eat with will make change a more palatable process.

Some of the lack of balance in your diet may be a result of where you are eating. Do you find yourself eating mindlessly while working at your computer or while watching TV? Do you automatically buy popcorn and soda when you go to a movie even if you've just finished dinner? Do you eat while you are driving? Are you even aware of the Calories that you are consuming while multitasking?

Take time now to make a list of all the places where you eat meals or snacks. Consider which of those places would be your choice for designated eating areas—locations that are appropriate for eating right. If you find you are overeating every time a food commercial comes on TV in the evening, then promise yourself that if you're hungry you will go into the kitchen and sit down to consume your snack. Plate the portion of the food you have picked so that you know how much you are going to eat, rather than eating right out of the box and losing track of what you've consumed.

How does your eating right help with balance in the world at large?

There are many implications for the environment and the economy in our food choices, not only in terms of how much we eat, but also in what we eat, where it comes from, and how many natural resources are consumed in the process. For those of you who have a backyard or even space on a balcony, I urge you to grow some herbs and vegetables or a tomato plant in a flowerpot. Not only will this enhance the types of food you buy at the market, but it also serves to connect what you eat with the source of your food. This can be part of living a whole life.

I challenge you to eat more whole foods that are unrefined or minimally processed. You will need to look beyond the front of the package when deciding if a food is "whole" or "whole grain." Even the nutrition facts on the label do not tell the complete story. You need to examine the ingredient list and look for the whole grain stamp on packages of truly whole grain breads and cereals. Some examples of whole grain foods are old-fashioned oatmeal and Shredded Wheat, which have only one ingredient and no additives. Ezekiel Bread and Alvarado Street Bakery Bread are examples of whole grain foods that are minimally processed. These are all low glycemic foods that tend to be more filling because of their high fiber content that results in the slow release of their carbohydrates.

Here is an example of a whole food continuum. Use this as a guide for what might be best for your body. The closer that you can stay to the left side, the better!

The Whole Food Continuum

Type of Food	Whole Food	Minimally Processed Food	Highly Refined Food
Oats	Steel Cut Oats	Oat Bran Muffin	Oat "O's" cereal
Wheat	Wheat Berries	Shredded Wheat	Wheat Flakes
Rice	Wild Rice	Brown Basmati rice	Instant Rice
Corn	Corn on the Cob	Cornmeal	Cornflakes
Pasta	Whole Wheat	Semolina Pasta	Couscous
Bread	Ezekiel Bread	Whole Wheat Bread	White Bread
Fruit	Fresh Pear	Canned Pears	Pear Nectar
Vegetable	Fresh Tomato	Canned Plum Tomatoes	Tomato Sauce

Maggie Davis

Week *7* Daily Devotionals

Theme for the Week # TRUST AND CORRECTION

Verse to Memorize *For the Lord disciplines him whom he loves, and chastises every son whom he receives.*

—HEBREWS 12:6

Day 1   The Restorative Power of Correction

R E A D | Galatians 6:1–10

Brethren, if a man is overtaken in any trespass, you who are spiritual should restore him in a spirit of gentleness. . . . Bear one another's burdens, and so fulfill the law of Christ. (vv. 1–2)

It comes as a distinct surprise to many Christians that they may have an obligation to correct other Christians, particularly those closest to them. This is so foreign to the experience most of us have in the church that this idea may seem to be a new or strange concept. Actually, the stranger concept is the idea that has slowly crept into our generation that we do *not* have responsibility for dealing with one another's faults. Minding one's own business, taking care only of one's self, turning a blind eye to the sins of our brothers and sisters—the Bible readings for this week will show us just how far these ideas are from the Gospel.

It is clear from the New Testament that being a Christian is about more than individual salvation. Yes, the Good Shepherd knows each of his sheep by name, but he has also placed each one into a flock. There, within the sheepfold, we learn how to love the Shepherd and how to love one another. We are responsible, according to the apostle Paul, to bear one another's burdens. At times, he says, this means "restoring" to the fellowship one who has "trespassed" into dangerous territory. This requires direct conversation (as we will see in later readings this week), for, if a person is in a fault or "trespass," how can he or she be "restored" unless the trespass is somehow addressed? How unloving is it to watch a fellow Christian do harm to him or herself and stand by doing nothing? God's word requires that we extend ourselves in love and in frankness for the sake of another.

Such a thing is almost unthinkable in today's church, except where groups of people covenant together—making a commitment of trust and love—to be honest with one another and to listen to one another. Certainly there is risk involved—hurt feelings, misunderstandings, fears about being so vulnerable with one another. Nevertheless, with the help of the Holy Spirit and the common wisdom of the group, such commitment leads to a depth of caring fellowship that can be the greatest blessing imaginable. This sense of investment in one another's lives is part of what it means to bear another's burden, and to bear our own load at the same time. The weight of responsibility to both give and receive correction lies squarely on our shoulders. It is a burden of love.

REFLECT | *What fears do you have when you consider this idea? What hopes? Some people are easier for you to be honest with than others are. Who is the hardest for you, and why?*

THOUGHT   ❝ Help me the slow of heart to move,
By some clear, winning word of love;
Teach me the wayward feet to stay,
And guide them in the homeward way. Amen. ❞
(Washington Gladden, 1836–1918)

Day 2   Face-to-Face

READ | Galatians 2
But when Cephas came to Antioch I opposed him to his face, because he stood condemned. (v. 11)

"Cephas" was Peter, the often brash and outspoken disciple of Jesus. Apparently, at this point in his life, he was having some difficulty living outwardly what he really believed in the face of opposition. In other words, he worried too much about what other people thought of him!

The situation is this: when Peter first came to Antioch, he mingled with the non-Jewish Christians and ate with them as equals. Then came "certain men from James," representing a group who felt that all Christians should be circumcised and strictly follow the Jewish rites.

This had become a point of serious controversy in the Jerusalem church, whose leaders were concerned when they heard that Paul was not requiring Gentiles to become Jewish proselytes when they became Christians. We know that Paul himself had been the strictest kind of Jew, and he knew from personal experience what observing the law meant. He also knew that God had generously thrown open the door of the kingdom to all people, both Jew and Gentile alike. So, when Peter saw the delegation from Jerusalem, he jumped up from the Gentile table and went over to a table made up of Jews only. Apparently, his fear of criticism led others to act just as "insincerely" (v. 13), and so Paul "opposed him to his face"—he confronted him with his hypocrisy.

This is a good example of how correction worked in the early church. The concern for truth and love was greater than the concern for personal opinions and feelings. For the sake of protecting and strengthening the fledgling body of Christ, face-to-face confrontation was often required. (Notice that Paul did not go away and complain to his fellow missionaries about Peter's actions.) The church will always be in need of such honest and loving people, for it will always be made up of sinners in need of the correcting influence of their brothers and sisters.

Of course, this commitment to honesty can sometimes be an excuse for erupting and dumping one's feelings on another out of jealousy, anger, or hurt feelings. But we have the same tools at our disposal that Paul had, in order to help prevent such abuses. First, we are committed to the overarching purpose of maintaining the "unity of the Spirit in the bond of peace" (Ephesians 4:3—more about this tomorrow). Essentially, this means that our primary goal is to love, not to harm, one another. And, second, we have Jesus' wise counsel to correct our "brother" (or sister) in the company of others (Matthew 18:15–16), and this is exactly what Paul did with Peter. With such tools at hand, what is there to keep us from correcting one another "face-to-face"?

REFLECT | *How does your worry about what others may think influence your actions? Be honest—what concerns you most: the need to be honest or the need to be understood? Why?*

Day 3   Telling the Truth: An Act of Love

READ | Ephesians 4

Therefore, putting away falsehood, let every one speak the truth with his neighbor, for we are members one of another. (v. 25)

As we are considering the subject of correction or reproof, it is good to prayerfully consider those places where we are "false" (that is, dishonest) in our relationships with fellow Christians. For example: Do we flatter insincerely? Do we, when recounting a story, alter the facts just enough to make ourselves look a little better? Do we pretend to approve of some attitude that we know to be wrong and hurtful? Do we indulge in hearsay and gossip, or enjoy listening to it a little too much, even if we do not repeat it? Do we harbor old resentments while outwardly acting as if we have forgiven?

The young church at Ephesus was in a hostile environment. At that time, Christians were often ostracized or directly persecuted for their faith. As we can see, Paul himself wrote this letter from prison. "I therefore, a prisoner for the Lord, beg you to lead a life worthy of the calling to which you have been called" (v. 1). His deep concern was

that the fellowship of Christians in Ephesus be *truthful* in all its attitudes and actions, lest it be sapped of the inner strength necessary to stand against all the outer forces that sought to destroy it.

Today, the church is still in great need of the spiritual reinforcement that is built when Christians "speak the truth in love" (v. 15). Paul tells us to be "eager" in our pursuit of unity and peace, but this does not mean a peace that comes at any price. He is essentially saying that the cost of the church's inner peace is its members' regular exchange of honesty and forgiveness. Nothing less will build up the church and make it "work properly" (v. 16). Nothing less will help its members to "grow up into Christ."

We cannot really know ourselves, nor fully know the ways of God, without the help of friends. In turn, we have an obligation of love that compels us to be truthful with those same friends. The church of Jesus Christ has been so conceived by heaven that its members need one another in this way. "Truth," wrote Henri-Frederic Amiel in the nineteenth century, "is the secret of eloquence and of virtue, the basis of moral authority; it is the highest summit of art and of life." Because the Cornerstone upon which the entire church is built is himself the Truth (John 14:6), is it any surprise that all its stones can adhere to one other only by living in the truth?

REFLECT | *Honestly consider the questions in the first paragraph. How would you answer them? Where recently have you been willing to speak the truth with your friends?*

THOUGHT ❝ Lord Jesus Christ, Keeper and Preserver of all things, let thy right hand guard us by day and by night, when we sit at home, and when we walk abroad, when we lie down and when we rise up, that we may be kept from all evil, and have mercy upon us sinners. Amen. ❞

(St. Nerses of Clajes, fourth century)

Day 4   Have I Become Your Enemy?

READ | Galatians 4:8–31

Have I then become your enemy by telling you the truth? (v. 16)

How well the Bible recognizes and describes the workings of human nature! When someone confronts us with an unpleasant truth about ourselves, don't we feel that this person is our enemy? (We certainly don't react this way to "pleasant truth"!) First, we often do not even recognize our friend's words as truth. It seems more like criticism, or condemnation, or even rejection. We find ourselves reacting with hurt—"How can she say such a thing?" We try defending ourselves—"You know I didn't mean it." Finally, we may get angry—"Who are you, anyway, to speak to me like that?" Whether or not we actually say these words makes no difference. When we feel "attacked," the person sitting across from us suddenly becomes our "enemy."

Paul knew that this was probably the way the Christians in Galatia were reacting to his correction. The whole letter is the stern but loving rebuke of one who had poured out his life to give these people the Good News of Jesus Christ. Now, he saw that they were in danger of selling their spiritual birthright for a mess of legalistic pottage, and he was angry! He was angry with those who had come into this young flock and unsettled their faith, and he was appalled at the Galatians themselves for being so gullible. His love for them led to one inevitable outcome: he must tell them the truth, unwelcome as it might be.

Paul knew that the light of truth always brings healing and stability.

But he also knew that his readers probably would not immediately welcome his honest words. When truth is spoken, it is often met with self-protective emotions. Still, truth is truth, and every hearer of the truth can choose to believe it, even though his or her feelings may go in exactly the opposite direction. After all, if we were ruled by our feelings alone, how stable could our faith be?

So, even though our emotions tell us that the person speaking to us is our "enemy," we can put our wills to work—we can choose to put down our defenses, we can listen carefully; we can pray for understanding; we can try to "agree with our adversary quickly" (see Matthew 5:25, KJV). Once we lay aside those defense mechanisms that we all use, we may be able to hear Paul's question as if it came from the mouth of the person speaking to us: "Have I become your enemy by telling you the truth?" "Of course not," we finally answer. And that is when the truth begins to set us free.

REFLECT | *When was the last time you treated a friend as an enemy? What things have you avoided saying because you were afraid someone would become angry with you?*

Day 5 Respect Those Who Admonish You

READ | 1 Thessalonians 5

But we beseech you, brethren, to respect those who labor among you and are over you in the Lord and admonish you, and to esteem them very highly in love because of their work. (vv. 12–13a)

Let's consider what the dictionary says about this word *admonish*: "to indicate duties or obligations to"; "to express warning or disapproval to, especially gently, earnestly, and solicitously"; "to give friendly, earnest advice or encouragement."

The word *admonish* comes from a word meaning "to warn." Those who admonish us are those who warn us of possible or real dangers in our lives, if we follow certain courses of action.

What role does admonishment play in the Christian's life? When someone asks for help, will you point out the "duties or obligations" that they must fulfill? When you see a brother or sister in need of correcting advice, are you willing to warn or disapprove, "gently, earnestly, and solicitously"? Are you open enough with your own struggles and temptations, so that others may give you "friendly, earnest advice or encouragement"?

Leaders, pastors, and others have a responsibility for those entrusted to their care, to give such help as they can. Earlier this week we read about Paul's admonishment of Peter. The Gospels are filled with examples of Jesus' admonishing words to his followers. The history of the church is replete with stories of the saints admonishing one another. All of us, without exception, need to be admonished from time to time. Without such words of "warning," "disapproval," and "advice," we risk the very grave danger of leaning on our own understanding and placing our own perceptions above those of all others. Such an attitude eventually breaks fellowship and separates us from those whom God has appointed to be our helpers in the faith—our families and other members of the body of Christ. You know how necessary it is, but also how difficult it can be, to admonish someone you love. Those who are willing to admonish you deserve your esteem and love, as well as your listening ear.

REFLECT | *What are some of the ways that others have admonished you? In what way do you see that they were speaking to you for God? Where have you cared enough for someone to offer admonishment?*

Day 6   The Rebuke of the Wise
[Just Tell Me the Truth]

READ | Ecclesiastes 7:1–20

It is better for a man to hear the rebuke of the wise than to hear the song of fools. (v. 5)

Who among us does not love to hear good things about him or herself? The self-affirming word is almost always the most welcome word. Making people feel better by saying good things about them is a popular remedy for gloom and discouragement, though its effects may actually be quite short-lived.

We all need to hear supportive, heartening words from friends and loved ones. In the Christian arsenal, encouragement is a strong weapon for successfully fighting off despair and sorrow. But we also must be fully aware that human nature's appetite for praise is voracious. Taking to oneself the glory that is due to God alone is an inherent aspect of sin, and it dwells in all of us. Seeking to "be like God" (as the book of Genesis describes the Fall, 3:5) has left us

with an unquenchable desire to be "loved, honored, worshiped, and adored." This is a far cry from the apostle Paul's frank admission that "nothing good dwells within me" (Romans 7:18). Perhaps Paul was echoing the words from Ecclesiastes in today's reading: "Surely there is not a righteous man on earth who does good and never sins" (v. 20).

How can we receive the honest correction of a friend if we only believe good about ourselves? Being realistic about ourselves—both about our desire for God as well as our penchant for sin—requires that we hear the bad with the good. "The rebuke of the wise" refers to something spoken out of a greater light than we have at the moment, a greater discernment and understanding than we have for ourselves. Most of us at times have such a word for others, and most of us have need of such a word from others. If we begin to see the love of God and the spirit of Jesus behind such words, then we can appreciate them for what they are—truths that are meant to penetrate our hearts and to change our lives.

Somerset Maugham once observed, "People ask you for criticism, but they only want praise." That may be well and good for the world apart from God. It is not well and good for Christians who are seeking to live their lives to the glory of God rather than to the glory of their own name. The songs that are sung to *our* praises are misdirected, and the one who listens too long to them is as foolish as the one who sings them.

REFLECT | *What do you believe about the role of correction in your own life? What is the purpose of an "encouraging word"?*

Day 7 A Sign of His Love

READ | Proverbs 3:1–12

My son, do not despise the LORD's discipline or be weary of his reproof, for the LORD reproves him whom he loves, as a father the son in whom he delights. (vv. 11–12)

We cannot be reminded enough times that the reproofs and corrections we receive from God are expressions of his immeasurable love for us. It is vitally important that we learn and hold fast to this truth as we go on following Jesus Christ. The writer of the Proverbs exhorts us to see God's hand of discipline as a hand of fatherly love and care for us. God "disciplines" us because he "delights" in us.

Most of us are newcomers to this concept. In adulthood, we may have accepted (even begrudgingly) that our parents did correct us in love, that they at least had our good in mind when they disciplined us, even if the means sometimes seemed severe or unfair. (This is not to excuse actual abuses. That is another matter altogether, and it can impair our vision of God as a genuinely loving father.) Furthermore, if we are parents ourselves, we know the motives we have for disciplining our children, even though we also know that parental correction is not always given without sin.

Still, it is better for a child to be corrected than not to be corrected, for his or her entire life will be shaped accordingly. To be sure, there are no sinless parents around, so we have to accept the fact that our parents did the best they knew and, before God, we can be grateful. At the same time, we can commit ourselves as parents to do the best we know, and to trust God with the results.

It goes without saying that, when discipline is given, no child welcomes it. The same can be said for the children of God. Even when we recognize the disciplining hand of God in our lives, we can still give way to self-pity and anger. We can grow "weary of his reproof." Self-pity says: "This is too much. I know I'm wrong, and I even know I need to change, but this is just not fair." Anger accuses: "How can you treat me this way? What did I do to deserve this?" This is precisely when we need to remember that God *never* corrects us outside of his love for us. His motives for disciplining us are never mixed. Pure love is all he can give!

REFLECT | *Where, in your life, have you seen that reproof and correction— either received or given—are expressions of loving concern?*

Week 8 Lifting the Burden of Guilt

The Plan

EATING RIGHT

- Try a new recipe from our website this week:
  www.3DYourWholeLife.com.

- Check your portions this week and see if you can
  cut down anywhere—a smaller piece of meat, a
  little less butter or salt, for example.

- Avoid eating while watching TV, working on the
  computer, or reading this week. See how this
  affects your eating.

LIVING WELL

- Do you stay up too late at night? Set a bedtime
  this week and see if you can add a half-hour
  more to your sleep time.

- Write a note or a letter to a friend or a family
  member this week just to let them know you are
  thinking about them.

- Count your steps. Are you meeting your goal?

LOVING GOD

- Read your daily devotions and memorize your
  new Scripture verse. Since we're talking about
  becoming free from guilt, if you have a setback
  this week, confess it to God and go on.

- Do not allow yourself to be discouraged, guilty,
  or angry. Every day *is* a new beginning.

Lifting the Burden of Guilt

THE GOOD NEWS OF THIS WEEK is that no matter where you've failed, or where you've gotten off course, God is waiting to take you and make something beautiful: the godly structure of mind, body, and spirit for which we were created.

Today I had a luncheon meeting with six other minister's wives. Just as in a 3D group, we meet regularly to talk and share and pray for each other. During the meeting, someone made a remark that hurt my feelings, and I knew I was shrinking inside. I had to make a choice: would I say anything or not? There was no question: I had to be honest. So I told the person how I felt when she said a certain thing. We discussed the incident, and I felt a sense of release. And all she had to do, after she realized what had hurt me, was to say, "I am sorry." My immediate response was, "I forgive you." Resolving that break in our relationship took less than five minutes, and we were able to practice again the lessons of God.

Openness, honesty, confession, forgiveness: what a wonderful process! Had I left that meeting without saying how I felt, I know beyond a doubt my feelings would have come out somewhere else, or I would have eaten the wrong thing just to make myself feel better. After thirty-five years, I know my habit patterns, and I must catch myself in order to keep from holding a grudge and being depressed. Guilt will weigh you down, while forgiveness will lift you up.

This week the theme is confession. Don't get caught up in feelings of guilt if you haven't kept to all of your original goals. God is there. The Holy Spirit of truth walks in our lives, through the words and actions of other people, and begins to set us free. Ask God to

Don't get caught up in feelings of guilt if you haven't kept to all of your original goals. God is there.

change your heart and to lift the burden of guilt you carry for not always achieving your goals. Accept God's forgiveness—and then be sure to forgive yourself. Say to God, "God help me. God forgive me. God, change my heart. Encourage me, dear Lord, to know that I am not who I can be, and in this process that I am in the middle of right now, I'm looking forward to becoming the woman or man that I want to be in my daily life."

THOUGHT 66 I am careful not to confuse
excellence with perfection.
Excellence, I can reach for;
perfection is God's business. 99

(Michael J. Fox, 1961–)

Excellence vs. Perfection

There is a big difference between striving for excellence and trying to be perfect. **Don't get caught up in perfection—not only is it bad for your spiritual life, but that's where the average diet fails.** If you focus on attaining a perfect body or reaching an ideal weight, you will be negative about who you are and where you are right now. You may avoid medical appointments for fear of being weighed on your doctor's scale. (That was Carol's experience.) You may be embarrassed when your doctor tells you for the umpteenth time to lose weight. You may have resorted to eating when you're alone. You may starve yourself every Monday but find that you binge by Thursday and then feel guilty about it.

Be your own Monday morning quarterback: review your food choices during the past week. Be honest with yourself, because by acknowledging what the problems are, you will be more able to develop a plan of action that works best for the next time. Rather than feeling guilty about a splurge or an impulsive restaurant choice, the secret of success in eating right for your whole life is to get back on track at your very next meal, rather than dwelling on your downfalls. That means that if you had a chocolate chip cookie at coffee break this morning, don't think that you've ruined your whole day of eating right. At lunch, perhaps you could leave one fourth of what you would usually eat, or you could have a smaller dinner that night to regain your balance.

A Nutritionist's Advice

Here are twelve basic strategies for eating right to lose weight:

- Break your fast every morning to rev up your metabolism early.
- Distribute food during the day in four to six meals or snacks.
- Consume more Calories during the day, less in the evening. Close the kitchen three hours before bedtime.
- Reduce saturated fat, animal fat, and refined carbohydrates. Replace them with foods made with whole grains, healthy oils, and less sugars.

- Meal replacements or portion-control packaged meals may be helpful. They may give you more control than leaving the house without eating or needing to stop for fast food.
- Portion control is an effective way to decrease Calories. Always decrease portions gradually to let your mind, body, and spirit adjust.
- Read labels before you buy (nutrition facts, ingredient lists, manufacturer's claims, and serving sizes). Consult a food composition book or a website for information about food that doesn't come with labels, such as fish, produce, or meat.
- Modify your usual recipes to make dishes healthier. Look for new ones that feature whole foods such as fruits, vegetables, whole grains, oils, and lean protein.
- Learn more about selecting, purchasing, storing, and preparing good quality foods. Spoiled food will not help your body or your wallet.
- Personalize your strategies for eating right. Find creative ways to gradually add healthy foods while decreasing less nutritious foods.
- Plan meals in advance whenever possible, but be prepared for changes, too.
- Track your intake of fiber, since it may reflect the overall wholeness of your diet.

Maggie Davis

Week 8 Daily Devotionals

Theme for the Week CONFESSION

Verse to Memorize *If we confess our sins,*
he is faithful and just,
and will forgive our sins
and cleanse us from
all unrighteousness.
—1 JOHN 1:9

Day 1 I Know My Transgression

READ | Psalm 51

Have mercy on me, O God, according to thy steadfast love; according to thy abundant mercy blot out my transgressions. Wash me thoroughly from my iniquity, and cleanse me from my sin! For I know my transgressions, and my sin is ever before me. (vv. 1–3)

The fifty-first Psalm is perhaps the greatest prayer of confession ever composed. We know the circumstances of its origin (see 2 Samuel 11 and 12), so we know that its words carry the heartfelt cry of one who was thoroughly convicted of his wrongdoing and deeply sorry for what he had done. Trusting only in the love of God, David threw open his soul before his Maker, and cast himself upon heaven's mercy. There is no better text to introduce this week's meditations on the combined subjects of repentance, confession, and forgiveness.

Jesus called the Holy Spirit, the "Spirit of truth" (John 16:13), telling his disciples that when the promised Spirit came, he would guide them into all truth. This includes the truth about themselves as well as the truth about God. The psalmist knew that, like a light shining in the darkness, God searches out our most inward being, and reveals to us our true condition. He, of course, knows it already. We are the only ones "in the dark" about ourselves.

Thank God that we have such an inward light, for we cannot repent if we do not know our transgression. Would a loving God leave us to our own blindness and self-delusion? As he did for King David, he desires that we "know our transgressions" so that we can also know his unfathomable mercy. Of course, as with the psalmist, it is not enough that we just talk about "mistakes" in our behavior. We are talking about the inward parts from which such behavior naturally springs—mixed motives, impure thoughts, jealous intentions, ruthless ambitions— these are among some of the dark places in the human soul.

When these things begin to come under the scrutiny of God, and the Spirit of truth begins to open our eyes to their presence, we squirm with discomfort and even denial. But keep this in mind: when a surgeon does his job, he has to know the specific details of both what and where the trouble is. Many of these details the patient might prefer to ignore if it were not for the disastrous consequences of such ignorance. Nonetheless, the immediate pain of knowing is far less than the future pain of not knowing. Knowing the truth about our condition is what leads to the joy of restoration and wholeness. This is an accurate picture of the process of conviction, repentance, and forgiveness. This is the message of Psalm 51.

REFLECT | *How would you describe your experience of the mercy of God? What are the "dark places" in your own life that the Holy Spirit has begun to illuminate for you? How are you responding to what he is showing you?*

Day 2   So Turn, and Live

READ | Ezekiel 18:21–32
*"For I have no pleasure in the death of anyone," says the Lord Go*D*, "so turn, and live." (v. 32)*

It is of the very nature of God to love, to give, and to be generous. He desires always to give life. After all, he is the Source of all life, and he created us to live with him forever. Death was never his intention for the human race (Genesis 3:17–19). Throughout both the Old and New Testaments, we see portrayed a God of mercy and patience, of forbearance and love—a God whose consuming interest is in whatever is best for his people. He desires life for us all!

It is a reassuring thought amidst the struggles of our lives, to know that God wishes always to impart life to us. Jesus said it in another way: "I came that they may have life, and have it abundantly" (John 10:10). In other words, his intent is for more than simply our existence. There is an overflowing fullness, a completeness, that he longs to give to his children.

What is it that hinders us from receiving that "abundant life"? Certainly not the purposes of God. It cannot be that God is unable to give what he wills to give. No force in heaven or earth can stay his hand. It must be that the obstacles to fully knowing God's abundant life lie within the receiver. Because of the unique place he has given humanity—made in the image of their Creator—he will not overrule or destroy our free wills. He will not make puppets of us. Instead, he allows us to stumble, to fall, to taste the fruit of our sinful choices, and to feel the pain of separation from him—to the end that we will turn back to him and live.

God sent the prophet Ezekiel to speak to the righteous as well as the wicked. The righteous he exhorts to keep to God's ways, lest they die. The wicked he implores to turn from their evil ways, and to live for God. This is the most basic meaning of repentance—to turn around and go the other way. Like the prophet, Jesus himself cried out to his people, "Repent, for the kingdom of heaven is at hand" (Matthew 4:17). Receiving the new life he comes to offer requires that we first turn away from the "old life." And this life of turning, of conversion—of having our minds and hearts re-formed into the likeness of Christ—is more than a one-time event. The Christian life involves turning, over and over again: when we have lapsed back into old, destructive patterns; when we have fallen to temptation; when we have willfully or ignorantly made choices to disobey God, the way is always open to us to turn around and go back to God. There we find him, with abundant life in his hands, ready to give it to us once again.

REFLECT | *What do you honestly believe about God's intent for you? In what ways is God asking you today to turn back to him? How can others be of help to you in your life of ongoing repentance?*

Day 3   No Longer Worthy
[Coming to Our Senses]

READ | Luke 15:11–32

But when he came to himself he said, "How many of my father's hired servants have bread enough and to spare, but I perish here with hunger! I will arise and go to my father, and I will say to him, 'Father, I have sinned against heaven and before you. . . .'" (vv. 17–18)

Jesus' parable of "the prodigal son" can be seen from a number of different points of view: the merciful patience and vigilance of the father; the self-assured independence of the young son; the jealous resentment of the elder brother; even the assumed wonder, perhaps confusion, of the servants. Certainly one of the story's most endearing qualities, however, is its portrayal of a young and foolish man's ambitions, of the depths to which he falls in order to keep to his stubborn ways, of his coming to his senses, and of his humble return to his father's house. As we consider the theme of confession this week, it is the young man's turnaround that we need to examine more closely.

First, his repentance came about when, having all that he held so dear stripped away, he came to the cold, hard realization of what he had done and of where his decisions had led him. "He came to himself," says Jesus (v. 17). We have explored this idea earlier this week—this process of facing what we have done and how we came to do it. His desperate circumstances served to remove the prodigal's self-protective blinders. He came to the painful realization that things were never going to get any better on the road he had chosen. So he chose a different path: "I will arise and go to my father."

Second, his confession was sincere and humble: "Father, I have sinned against heaven and before you; I am no longer worthy to be called your son." Finding his father waiting on the road for his return, he might have been tempted to avoid that painful admission. But the young man knew what he had to say. He had to acknowledge with his lips the dreadful truth that he knew about his life.

Finally, the young man's repentance and confession opened

the way to forgiveness and joy. The forgiveness of his father was a free gift, but he would never have been in the place to receive that gift had he not "come to himself" and returned home. This is the way it is with God and his sons and daughters. His arms are always ready to embrace us when we are ready to repent. His heart is always ready to welcome us when we are ready to confess. His love is always ready to forgive us when we are ready to receive. Like the prodigal son, all we need do is come to our senses.

REFLECT | *In what ways has God helped you to "come to your senses" when you have wandered from his ways? What people or circumstances might God be using today to bring you back to himself?*

Day 4   Confess Your Sins to One Another

READ | James 5

Therefore confess your sins to one another, and pray for one another, that you may be healed. (v. 16)

In recent weeks, we have explored the issue of truthfulness and openness in our relationships with other Christians, particularly those with whom we are covenanted together in love. Today we touch upon a crucial aspect of that openness—confession. James tells us that confession of our sins to one another brings healing and peace. A question and a caution are in order at this point. The question: when should we confess our sins to another person? The Bible puts no limit on the practice. It is *always* appropriate to admit our sin to another. However, this brings us to the caution: certainly it is unwise to make certain confessions—like sexual misconduct or similarly intimate and sensitive sins—to anyone other than a trustworthy pastor, priest, or mature counselor.

Having said that, however, there are countless sins of both attitude and action that we can and should confess to other Christians—to members of a prayer group, or wherever God has provided people willing to "bear one another's burdens, and so fulfill the law of Christ." Sometimes confessing our sins privately to God does not seem to bring relief from the burden or guilt, and we need additional help from others, face-to-face. Here, the words of the German pastor Dietrich Bonhoeffer apply:

> God has willed that we should seek and find his living word in the witness of a brother, in the mouth of a man. Therefore, the Christian needs another Christian who speaks God's word to him. He needs him again and again when he becomes uncertain and discouraged, for by himself, he cannot help himself without belying the truth. He needs his brother man as a bearer and proclaimer of the divine word of salvation.

That "word of salvation" is often the assurance of forgiveness after we have exposed to others our jealousy or anger, our rebellion or resentment. That we are loved and accepted, forgiven and cleansed, even when we are blatantly wrong (*especially* when we are blatantly wrong), is a reason for much rejoicing for the sinner and for the entire fellowship. That "word of salvation" may also be additional insight into the problem we are confessing, as we come to see more clearly that we are often behaving out of subconscious, perhaps unhealed, feelings and motivations. Once these dark places within us are brought "into the light," they often lose their hold on us, and our confessors become the instruments of God's healing peace in our lives.

REFLECT | *James tells us clearly that we should confess our sins to others— what makes this difficult to do? Describe a time when you experienced the joy of forgiveness and the peace of restored relationships after confessing your sin.*

THOUGHT

❝ My God is reconciled;

His pard'ning voice I hear;

He owns me as his child;

I can no longer fear.

With confidence I now draw nigh,

And, "Father, Abba, Father," cry! ❞

(Charles Wesley, 1707–1788)

Day 5 When God Convicts, Do We Act?

READ | Jonah 3

When God saw what they did, how they turned from their evil way, God repented of the evil which he had said he would do to them; and he did not do it. (v. 10)

The city of Nineveh was renowned for its wickedness. God's word came to the prophet Jonah, saying, "Arise, go to Nineveh, that great city, and cry against it; for their wickedness has come up before me" (1:2). This divine intervention sets the stage for the events that follow.

There was no doubt about Nineveh's need for repentance. But there is an unusual feature to this story. Apparently, Jonah's instruction was only to "cry out" against Nineveh's sin and to declare its impending doom. There was no direct call for repentance as such. It would be up to the citizens of the city to decide what to do—if anything— with the prophet's message.

This story can give us some clues as to how God sometimes gets our attention and addresses our sin. For example, certain distressing circumstances or seemingly insoluble problems that we cannot avoid may come into our lives. Or, within our own souls there may arise a feeling of unsettledness, or anxiety, or even guilt. Or, a friend or a family member may be hurt or angry with us for something we have done and cannot undo. It is not always the case that God is using these events to tell us that we are wrong about something and we do not know it, but it is worth prayerfully pursuing the question. Instead, what is our usual response to such things: Anger? Self-defense? Hurt? Withdrawal?

A good example of what *not* to do in such circumstances is seen in 1 Samuel 3. Young Samuel received a message to deliver to Eli, the priest, warning of God's judgment upon Eli's house because of his sons' wickedness. Eli's answer?—"It is the LORD; let him do what seems good to him" (1 Samuel 3:18). Resigned to his fate, the man made no effort whatsoever to change.

The people of Nineveh were wiser. Though the prophet held out no hope for their salvation, the king declared, "Let everyone turn from his evil way. . . . Who knows, God may yet . . . turn from his fierce anger" (vv. 8–9). (Even the animals were dressed contritely in sackcloth!) The implication here is that God means his word—however it comes to us—to convict us of our wrong and to lead us to genuine repentance. Our task is to listen carefully for that word, and then to act upon it.

REFLECT | *If you are truly sorry for your sin, you will want to change. What specific steps are you taking to allow God to change you? What is the difference between remorse and repentance?*

Day 6 Purified by Blood

READ | Hebrews 9

Without the shedding of blood there is no forgiveness of sins. (v. 22b)

The entire Old Testament sacrificial system begins to make sense when we see it as a foreshadowing of what one hymn-writer called the "one, true, pure immortal sacrifice" of Jesus Christ (William Bright, 1874). The blood—that is, the "life"—of bulls and lambs and goats was shed in anticipation of the Lamb of God who would take away the sin of the world (John 1:29).

What does that mean for the Christian? First, it means that the shedding of Jesus' blood is a pure sacrifice for our sin, and that forgiveness and remission are applied when that sin is "washed . . . in the blood of the Lamb" (Revelation 7:14). God has freely given the soul-cleansing blood of his Son to free us from the stain and pollution of sin. It is his divine solution to the problem of human sin, from the sin of Adam and Eve right on down to the sin you and I will commit today. The blood of Christ is sufficient to purify us all.

Practically speaking, however, we can know that cleansing power only as we face our sin head-on, confess it, and seek God's forgiveness. As we will read tomorrow in the first letter of John: "If we walk in the light, as he is in the light, we have fellowship with one another, and the blood of Jesus his Son cleanses us from all sin" (1:7). Notice what the apostle says: it is when we are living "in the light," attempting neither to hide our wrong nor to justify it, that the cleansing power of Christ's blood takes effect. He goes on to warn: "If we say we have not sinned, we make him a liar, and his word is not in us" (v. 10).

This makes clear that the honest acknowledgment and confession of our sin is an essential part of the cleansing and healing process.

Second, the shedding of Christ's blood means that our good works cannot make up for our wrongs. From God's point of view, we have no righteousness of our own to offer for the salvation of our souls. As Paul writes, "None is righteous, no, not one" (Romans 3:10). Still, even after we have tasted God's forgiving love, we are prone to fall back into the old and useless pattern of trying to compensate for our wrongness by doing good or right things. Such acts may make us feel better for a time, but they will never make recompense for our sin. The Bible makes it clear: the stain of sin is removed through confession and forgiveness—not through working harder at being right. True "good works" can be born only out of gratitude for God's salvation and obedience to his will. If we ever think that our own goodness is sufficient to see us through, then we are "in the dark" about our own desperate need, and we slander the "one, true, pure, and immortal sacrifice" of our Savior.

REFLECT | *What does the sacrifice of Jesus Christ mean to you personally? Where have you recently tried to "make up" for your wrong: Before others? Before God?*

Day 7   He Will . . .

READ | 1 John 1

He is faithful and just, and will forgive our sins and cleanse us from all unrighteousness. (v. 9)

George Adam Smith wrote, "The forgiveness of God is the foundation of every bridge from a hopeless past to a courageous present." This is what we all long for: a "courageous present"—a present that is as free as possible from fears and anxieties, from destructive habits, and from worn-out ways of reacting to people and circumstances. No, we have not yet arrived at that "courageous present," we are not yet whole, we are not yet at perfect peace—but we are on the way.

At the end of this week, it is important to ask once again, "Why this emphasis upon confession, repentance, and forgiveness?" We might even add, "I am a committed Christian. I know that Jesus forgave me for my sins when I accepted him as my Savior, and I know that he has

cleansed me from the past. What is confession about now?"

There is no doubt about it. If we know the saving love of Jesus Christ, then we also know that our lives have been made new. *But* (and this is an inescapable "but"), we also know that we are still faced with our*selves*—expressions of the same "old self" that keep popping up and disturbing us all along our way. Having given our lives to Christ with all our hearts, some of us become discouraged by our ongoing failure to be faithful to the ways in which we know we should live. The sense of victory that once filled our hearts has given way to the nagging feeling of defeat. Some become so disheartened by this onslaught of their "old nature" (Ephesians 4:22) that they settle for "pretending"—doing everything in a Christian manner on the outside, while their faith decays from within. Some are tempted to give up their faith altogether.

This short chapter from the first letter of John is the answer to this dilemma. What is born of God, the life of the Holy Spirit within us, *is* of God. *We* are of God. This is an irrefutable reality for every child of God—Christ is in us. Equally true, however, is that the old nature, what the apostle Paul calls "sin which dwells within me" (Romans 7:17), is also there, seeking to express itself in all its old, familiar ways. God has provided a way out of this conflict, and it is available to us every day!—"If we confess our sins, he is faithful and just, and will forgive our sins and cleanse us from all unrighteousness." The day will come when the victory won for us by the Cross and Resurrection of Jesus Christ will be completely fulfilled. Until that final day comes, do not despair. We can have a foretaste of that victory every day of our lives— through repentance, confession, and forgiveness.

REFLECT | *Name some times, perhaps recently, when you were tempted to be discouraged about the quality of your Christian life. What helped you to renew your strength? What does it mean to you to be forgiven?*

Week 9 Understanding Your Emotions

The Plan

EATING RIGHT

▦ Record your emotions this week as you eat, paying special attention to the patterns and trends that you see.

▦ List three trigger foods and the emotions or circumstances that are occurring when you eat them.

▦ Identify the major stress factors in your life this year, and write them in your journal.

LIVING WELL

▦ Try one or more of these non-food options for coping with negative feelings:

  ▪ Call a friend.
  ▪ Go outside at night to look at the stars and the heavens.
  ▪ Buy yourself some flowers or pick some wildflowers.
  ▪ Listen to soothing music to change your mood.
  ▪ Take a shower or a bath.
  ▪ Go for a short walk.
  ▪ Take a nap, or simply put your feet up.
  ▪ Start your own list.

▦ Increase your daily steps by 100.

LOVING GOD

▦ This week, pray and meditate on your Scripture verse outdoors. Experience God in the trees, mountains, sunset, or rivers, and feel his light and blessing.

Understanding Your Emotions

THIS IS A MOST DELICATE SUBJECT FOR ME. I am a very emotional person. I wear my feelings on my sleeve. And I know that many of my eating habits are directly related to my emotions. Much of the time when I eat I am not even sure I am hungry. I do know I am angry, or I am hurt, or I am sad, or I am jealous. I am very much in touch with both my negative and positive feelings. However, cutting the connection between those feelings and what I put in my mouth is not always easy.

For many years, I had no idea that my compulsive eating was related to my feelings. Nowadays there are many magazine articles that say it in black and white: deal with your feelings and you will deal with your weight. I just wish that knowing all of those facts and even believing them would have healed me completely. But the battle goes on.

The good news is that I am now more in charge of those feelings, and they don't run me as they have in years past. The bad news is that an ice cream cone on a beautiful summer evening still makes me feel better! (Sorry, Maggie!) But now this is a choice I make consciously; now it is not a undisclosed negative feeling or a bad habit that "makes" me eat the ice cream. And then immediately I can jump back on the "eat right" campaign.

We should not consider some emotions as being good and some as being bad. For example, some of us think that crying about a death is acceptable, but crying about a fear is not, thus making one a positive expression and one a negative one. Emotions simply express feelings. We must not sift through them when they

> We should not consider some emotions as being good and some as being bad.

arise, and then decide if it is indeed safe to express them. We need to face them, talk about them, express them, and determine whether they will continue the process of making us whole, or whether they will be destructive in this process. Emotions surface whether we want them to or not. They are part of who we are even if we hide them.

Many years ago, I attended the funeral of a sixteen-year-old boy. My understanding of God changed in that funeral service because of a song that was sung, "There's a Wideness in God's Mercy." One of the verses says this:

> There is no place where Earth's sorrows
>> are more felt than up in Heaven.
> There is no place where Earth's failings
>> have such kindly judgment given.

It was at that moment that I realized that God does not sit on a throne looking down at life's tragedies and asking me to ignore them. He wants me to face how I feel; he wants to walk me through those hard places. Those few words—"There is no place where Earth's sorrows are more felt than up in Heaven"—helped me recognize that my deep sorrow had, and has, its rightful place in my Christian life.

There was no way I could put wonderful spiritual terms on this painful event, the funeral of a teenager. I had many more questions than I had answers, and I was dreading going through the process of facing the young man's mom and dad and saying empty words, such as "God must have needed him more in heaven." I was sad and even mad at the useless loss of a beautiful life. However, standing in that church and singing that song let me know that God was feeling this sorrow even more than we were on earth. I have no idea what that means theologically. I just saw tears in God's eyes that day, and knew I was beginning a new relationship with a God who understands sadness and sorrow.

THIS EXPERIENCE LET ME KNOW THAT GOD must also understand my own anger and hurt and pain, and that I can tell him exactly how I feel and seek his help to get me out of those dark, hard places. I must not dwell in those feelings and make myself miserable. God wants to help me through my pain. It is okay to have emotions, even if they are negative. The power of them is released once we talk about them.

Now my prayer is that God will use the emotional woman that I am in a constructive way to understand, to empathize with, to communicate with, and to love those around me. This week, you will begin to recognize your emotions, positive or negative, and you will be encouraged to ask God to help you not to be controlled by them. Get to know your emotions this week. Only then can your whole life really come into balance.

Emotional Triggers

Bet you can't eat just one!
(Lay's Potato Chip advertisement)

One day last summer, I had a follow-up appointment with a wonderful woman named Roberta to discuss her diet and her progress controlling her Type 2 Diabetes. Roberta told me that it had taken her longer than usual that day to drive to my office. When I asked why, she said that she had had to take a longer route to avoid a hot dog vendor who was positioned along her usual route. "My steering wheel starts to pull my car over when I see the sign for hot dogs," she said, and so for the entire summer she chose to avoid the vendor completely.

Roberta was successful in avoiding a food that has always been a temptation for her. In time, she may be able to take the shorter route to my office—but for now, her strategy is working just fine! She was able to understand that her childhood pleasure in having a hot dog during the summer was no longer serving her need to control her diabetes.

In the second third of the 3D plan, you laid many of the building blocks for creating a new way of eating right. By now, you have adjusted the quality of your daily intake and decreased your portions of some foods, and increased your intake of vegetables. Each person works on these issues at his or her own pace.

As you have been recording your daily diet, you have also started to record some of the feelings that are associated with your eating habits and food choices. During the course of keeping your journal, **you may have noticed that certain foods may serve as a trigger for you to eat more.** These are often highly processed foods with ingredients that actually stimulate your appetite. They may contain salt, fat, and sugar in some combination. Some of them may even be marketed as "diet foods." Sometimes they are favorite foods such as ice cream or watermelon that taste so cool and refreshing on a hot day that you just keep eating them without considering the Calories or your fullness level. These trigger foods are generally quick to eat and require little or no preparation. Or they may simply be available, like the roast or casserole you prepared that is sitting on the stove with more available to eat after dinner. Make notes in your journal when this happens so that you can identify the food involved as well as your emotional state or stress level at the time. This will help you to identify foods that you may want to avoid completely, since simply having one bite seems to create a craving for more.

The following factors can contribute to compulsive eating—be on the watch for these in yourself and in other members of your 3D group:

- Unexpressed anger or other strong emotions
- Despair, sadness, or grief
- A feeling of worthlessness or helplessness
- Loneliness or isolation
- The feeling that extra weight may serve as a protection against getting hurt again
- Past or present emotional or physical abuse
- Acute stress

In some cases, binge-eating that is caused by emotional triggers is best treated through counseling or therapy.

Use Your Emotions to Eat Well

Start to note your emotions this week as you eat. Think about (and record) how you feel each time you have a meal, a snack, or a taste of food. Reflect on what you've eaten. Examine your journal and reflect on the patterns and trends that you see. If you recognize in the course of recording that you are eating for emotional reasons, you may already have identified the feelings you are experiencing. **Be as specific as you can in describing the feeling you are having.** Does eating really help you feel better for very long? Or does emotional eating make you feel even more guilt and shame?

This week focus your journal on these unpleasant feelings that surface. By recording them, you are accepting that they exist. That's the first step toward coping with them. As you find yourself turning to food for emotional reasons, assuming that you are not experiencing physical hunger, try first taking a "time out." (Yes, those things we use with our toddlers sometimes make sense for us, too!) Step away from the refrigerator or the kitchen or the convenience store. Take a few minutes to relax by doing some deep, focused breathing. Sit quietly with your feet on the floor, and with your mouth closed, take a long, slow breath, filling your lungs completely. Then slowly breathe out through your mouth. As you repeat these steps, concentrate on relaxing your muscles, your mind, and your heart. You will find that the more you practice taking time out, the more quickly you will be able to relax.

Next, take a few moments to think about other alternatives to eating. (But do this *second*, not *first*.) What would be a smarter choice to help cope with these feelings? **I recommend that you start to develop a list or a repertoire of non-food de-stressors that you can turn to, when in the past you might have overeaten.** Include positive things you can do for yourself.

Maggie Davis

Week 9 Daily Devotionals

Theme for the Week EMOTIONS

Verse to Memorize   *If we confess our sins,*
he is faithful and just,
and will forgive our sins
and cleanse us from
all unrighteousness.
—1 JOHN 1:9

Day 1   The Anger and Sorrow of God

READ | Genesis 6:1–8; Deuteronomy 9:13–29

And the LORD was sorry that he had made man on the earth, and it grieved him to his heart. (Genesis 6:6)

And the LORD was so angry with Aaron that he was ready to destroy him. (Deuteronomy 9:20)

This week, we are tackling a sizable subject—our emotions: oh, how they trouble us and please us, invigorate us and distress us . . . and those around us, as well. How do they fit into our lives of discipleship? What can we or should we be doing about them? How can they both serve us and shackle us in our relationships with God and with one another?

As we begin this exploration, it is important that we remember that our emotions are part of what links us with our Creator. The Bible says that we have been made in the image of God. The Bible also describes God, especially in his incarnate Son, Jesus Christ, as having a whole range of emotions: anger, sorrow, joy, peace. We do not read that God is placid and numb, dwelling always in eternal calm. God's "emotions," of course, are untainted by sin. They are not provoked by fear or anxiety, by resentment or surprise. Still, their

presence is indisputable. So, even though we cannot fully understand how it is that a changeless God can "feel" delight or displeasure, we can know that the feelings we have are in some way connected to our heavenly origins. Perhaps knowing this can help us to better accept our emotional make-up, while, at the same time, it can teach us that our emotions, like the rest of our *selves*, must be brought under the dominion of God.

Consider today's readings. They tell us that God knows both sorrow and anger, sometimes amongst the most difficult emotions for us to express. What are some of the things that bring sorrow to God? "Woe to those," says the prophet Amos, "who lie upon beds of ivory, and stretch themselves upon their couches, and eat lambs from the flock . . . sing idle songs . . . drink wine in bowls, and anoint themselves with the finest oils, but are not grieved over the ruin of Joseph!" (Amos 6:4–6). The ruin of his people, the sin that blemishes and deforms his creation, the ongoing rebellion of humanity and its disastrous consequences— these bring grief and sorrow to the Father's heart. What makes God angry? In the reading for today, it is clear that the natural tendency of the people to trample underfoot the gifts of God—the miracles of the Passover, the parting of the Red Sea, and all the other divine deliverances—and to turn away to their own inventions: these are the things that kindle the just anger, the righteous wrath of a Holy God.

Take heart. If the Creator of the universe is, himself, familiar with even these strong emotions of sorrow and anger, can we not trust that he also knows our own, and that he knows how to help us live with them?

REFLECT | *What emotions in yourself are you the most afraid or resistant to express? Why? What emotions in others make you the most nervous? Why?*

Day 2   The Joy of the Almighty

READ | Isaiah 62

As the bridegroom rejoices over the bride, so shall your God rejoice over you. (v. 5)

Joy is one of those emotions that we most *enjoy*, and that we probably wish we experienced more often. There is a natural tenseness that comes from living in a fallen world, and our cynical generation seems more adept than ever at smothering joy and enticing us to find it in false places. Still, the ability to rejoice is commensurate with our wholeness in the Lord. Someday, our joy will be unbounded in its fullness and unfettered in its expression. Until that time, how do we have more of it?

The Scriptures urge us: "Rejoice always" (1 Thessalonians 5:16); "Rejoice in the Lord always; again I will say, Rejoice" (Philippians 4:4); and "Rejoice and be glad" (Psalm 118:24). This is easier said than done, we say. However, as we discussed yesterday, it is helpful to know that God himself experiences joy. Perhaps we can learn more about what brings us joy by understanding more about what brings God joy.

In his job as God's spokesman, the prophet Isaiah was often burdened with a very difficult responsibility—bringing *bad news* to his king and his people: "I will turn my hand against you"; "I will break down your walls"; "I will turn your springs into deserts." But in the last half of the book of Isaiah, he is most often the deliverer of *good news*: "I will make your ways straight"; "I will comfort your sorrows"; "I will rejoice in Jerusalem and be glad in my people." We know at least three things from all these declarations of God's joy:

First, God rejoices out of love for his people. The imagery of these words in chapter 62 is that of the relationship between a bridegroom and his bride. The essential ingredient in that relationship is love. Joy and love are emotional siblings, and this means that giving and receiving love will always bring us joy.

Second, God rejoices when what he knows is best for his people is accomplished in their lives. God's joy and God's will are inseparably entwined. Jesus found delight in doing the will of his Father. Does this not tell us one place to locate the spring from which we might draw our own joy?

Finally, God rejoices in all his works, and you and I are among them. The good things he has done, and is still doing, in our lives are all reasons for rejoicing. When God is at work, we do well to try to see things from his point of view, for what he sees is good.

Yes, there are innumerable reasons to be glum and downhearted. But there are more reasons to give thanks and rejoice. It is essential to our wholeness in Christ that we learn to cultivate the emotion of joy—not a joy that is shallow or phony, but a joy that is deeply rooted in the love, the will, and the goodness of God.

REFLECT | *What has God done, or is he now doing, in your life that brings you joy? It is often the case that by suppressing or indulging in our negative emotions, we end up suppressing our joy as well. Where is this true in your life?*

THOUGHT **❝** Be happy. Be content—always, everywhere, in all circumstances—because every circumstance is a gift of love for you from the Eternal Father. That's why God wants us to rejoice in every one of our troubles, and to praise and give glory to His name—yes, in everything—because God loves you with a forever kind of love.

Buck up! Remember who loves you, and be encouraged today and every day in Christ, gentle Jesus. **❞**

(Catherine of Siena, 1347-1370)

Day 3   A Man of Sorrows

READ | John 11:1–44

When Jesus saw her weeping, and the Jews who came with her also weeping, he was deeply moved in spirit and troubled; and he said, "Where have you laid him?" They said to him, "Lord, come and see." Jesus wept. (vv. 33–35)

The prophet Isaiah called God's Suffering Servant "a man of sorrows, and acquainted with grief" (Isaiah 53:3). Did he have some preview into the tearful grief of the Son of Man? Referring to the passage in John 11, one writer asks, "Is it for nothing that the Evangelist, some sixty years after it occurred, holds up to all ages, with such touching brevity, the sublime spectacle of the Son of God in tears? What a seal of his perfect oneness with us in the most redeeming feature of our stricken humanity. . . . The tears of Mary and her friends acted sympathetically upon him, and drew forth his emotions. What a vivid outcoming of real humanity!"

Knowing that we have a great High Priest who is able "to sympathize with our weaknesses"

(Hebrews 4:15), we should never be reticent or ashamed to face our own feelings of frailty, sorrow, grief, or loneliness. These are the emotions that we often try to deny, or at least keep under control. But what do we do with this picture of Jesus, standing before the people he loved, making no effort whatsoever to hide his sorrow or hold back his tears?

Jesus Christ is the image of a perfected humanity. When confronted with the bitter loss of his friend and the mournful faces of those most dear to him, he wept. Apparently, wholeness and maturity have nothing to do with stoicism and reserve. Yet, for some reason, most of us are uncomfortable with our own sorrow and, therefore, with the sorrow of others. A man told me once that, as a child, he used to bite his tongue until it bled in order to keep from crying. What is it that compels us to hold back such emotions? Sometimes it is the example of others; sometimes it is our own pride, and our need to always look strong and "put together"; sometimes it is the fatalistic and self-protective echo in our brains that says, "crying about it won't do any good anyway."

However, to deny such emotions is to deny our linkage with the Son of Man himself. Crying may not *solve* the problem, but it is certainly a step toward acknowledging that there *is* a problem, and that is often the first step to healing. Genuine sorrow is a sign that we are genuinely human. The joyful day will come when God will wipe every tear from our eyes, and when there will be no more crying or pain (Revelation 21:4). In the meantime, we can know the sympathy of the Man of Sorrows, and that is no small comfort.

REFLECT | *What feelings do you consider "unacceptable" and therefore seek to suppress? Unexpressed sorrow can actually twist itself into other forms: bitterness, fear, or aloofness, for example. What is your experience?*

Day 4   Be Angry but Do Not Sin

READ | Ephesians 4:17–32

Be angry but do not sin; do not let the sun go down on your anger. (v. 26)

In a single line, the apostle Paul touches upon two aspects of anger: anger that is justified, and anger that can be destructive. In the case of justifiable anger, Charles Haddon Spurgeon, the great nineteenth-century English preacher, has this word to say: "Anger is not always or necessarily sinful, but it has such a tendency to run wild that whenever it displays itself we should be quick to question its character with this enquiry: 'Doest thou well to be angry?' It may be that we can answer, 'Yes.' Very frequently anger is the madman's firebrand, but sometimes it is Elijah's fire from heaven. We do well when we are angry with sin, because of the wrong it commits against our good and gracious God; or with ourselves, because we remain so foolish after so much divine instruction; or with others, when the sole cause of anger is the evil they do. He who is not angry at transgression becomes a partaker in it."

Paul makes a differentiation between being angry and sinning.

There are some things that we *should* be angry about! But many of us think of anger as always being wrong and ugly (and most of us strive so hard *never* to be wrong and ugly), so we repress the anger that rises up within us and try to deny its undeniable existence! Yet, it may be "righteous anger," a justifiable reaction to sin and the harm that it is causing in someone else's life.

Of course, it is obvious that anger does have its downside, and Paul has something to say about that as well. The J.B. Phillips translation puts the verse this way: "If you are angry—be sure that it is not out of wounded pride or bad temper. Never go to bed angry—don't give the devil that sort of foothold."[3] Anger that goes unexamined and unchecked can turn into a destructive plaything for the devil, disturbing our own peace of mind as well as the peace that should prevail in our relationships. Whatever you do, says Paul, do not end the day in anger.

Once we know that we are angry, it is up to us—prayerfully, and often with the help of friends—to discover the source of that anger. On the one hand, if we find that our anger is springing forth from our own sin—such as hurt pride, jealousy, or fear of losing control—we need to be quick about confessing it and seeking its remedy. On the other hand, if we find that its cause is a genuine concern for others, or real pain caused by others, then we cannot hesitate to let it be known. In any case, we must accept the fact that anger is a part of our essential emotional make-up. We cannot avoid it. More than likely, we will discover that we have a fair amount of bottled-up anger that we have admitted neither to ourselves nor to others. This might be the time to be honest about it.

REFLECT | *List some of the things that make you angry. What is the source of those angers? What do you do with your anger? Sometimes we use our anger—either spoken or unspoken—to control others. Can you identify any places in your life where this is true for you?*

Day 5   When I Am Afraid

READ | Psalms 55, 56
When I am afraid, I put my trust in thee. (56:3)

Fear is one of the basic emotions common to all humans. In fact, fear is an emotion we share with all creatures. It serves a critical purpose—warning us of danger, rousing us to greater effort under stress, and correcting our inclination to negligence or foolishness. A healthy amount of fear is essential to our well-being.

Moreover, we are told that "the fear of the LORD is the beginning of wisdom" (Proverbs 9:10). A holy fear of God—knowing that he is our Maker and that he holds our lives accountable before his righteous judgment: this kind of fear is both prudent and productive. Without it, it is doubtful that we would be moved toward any kind of obedience at all.

Few if any of us can claim that our desire to do God's will stems only from our love for him.

Yet, the Bible also tells us that "perfect love casts out fear" (1 John 4:18). Fear has the potential of growing beyond its proper and useful function, and can distort itself into a paralyzing and devastating emotion. Fear then becomes our mortal enemy. ("We have nothing to fear but fear itself," said President Franklin Roosevelt.) In the hands of the devil, and fed by the unhealed areas of our own lives, fear can enslave us within its chains of faithlessness, sapping our energy, undermining our hopes, and distracting us from the goal set before us. It can set us at enmity with others and blind us to the love of God. The psalmist was well acquainted with the gripping force of fear. He writes, "The terrors of death have fallen upon me. Fear and trembling come upon me, and horror overwhelms me" (55:4–5). Surrendering to fear, when it reaches such inordinate proportions, can have tragic results.

So, what is the solution? First, do not deny the presence of fear. This is always the first step in overcoming it. Look at how honest the psalmist was about his own fears. "*When* I am afraid," he said. Not *if*, but *when*. One of the most dangerous and foolish things we can do is pretend to be brave when we are not! Fear can never—*never*—be controlled in that way. Once you acknowledge its grip on you, bring it before God in honest confession. Just as the psalmist did, ask him for his help and deliverance. Consider admitting your fear to a friend, to someone you trust. Perhaps together, you can find its cause or, at the very least, see it for what it really is.

Our fears prevail over us because our faith is so weak within us. The antidote to fear is "perfect love," meaning that, in coming to know the limitless and ever-present love of God for us, and to love him in return, we grow strong in our trust. "When I am afraid," writes the psalmist, "I put my trust in thee. . . . in God I trust without a fear" (Psalm 56:3–4). We can move from fear to faith—over and over again, because we can trust in God, who loves us and who intends nothing but what is best for us.

REFLECT | *Being as honest as you can be, list the fears in your life. Do you know the root cause of any of them? What are they? Choose one, and prayerfully think about how you can move it from fear to faith.*

Day 6   Learning to be Genuine

READ | Romans 12

Let love be genuine; hate what is evil, hold fast to what is good; love one another with brotherly affection; outdo one another in showing honor. (vv. 9–10)

This week we are discussing our emotions, placing a good deal of emphasis on the need to face them as authentic and necessary (albeit, at times, confusing and unruly) parts of our lives. Hiding them, suppressing them, denying them— these are among the least productive ways of living with our emotions. If truthfulness—genuineness—is one mark of the Christian, then it must apply as much to our feeling as it does to our thinking.

One of the prime purposes— perhaps *the* prime purpose—of the Christian life is to glorify God. In other words, our purpose is to have our lives perfectly reflect their Maker and conform to the divine intentions for which they were created—to become God-centered instead of self-centered, to love God and neighbor with all our hearts, and in every way to be like Jesus. A great teacher and leader of the second-century church, Irenaeus, wrote: "The glory of God is humanity, fully alive." *Fully alive.* Isn't this the longing of our hearts? Of course, sin enters the picture here, and it fractures every aspect of that longed-for fullness of life, including our emotions. Therefore, we can know the wholeness God intends for us only as the Holy Spirit does his healing work in our lives. God puts the pieces back together, in their proper places and with their proper functions, the way he created them to be in the first place.

Among the things "fractured" by sin are relationships, together with all the emotions that weave through them. The twelfth chapter of Romans addresses this all-important aspect of Christian fellowship. Paul recognizes that forces exist, both outside and inside, that undermine the unity of this fellowship. For example, he says, "Do not be conformed to this world," because he knows that the world's values contradict the values of heaven. We are to live differently.

We contend against inner forces as well. For example, Paul writes: "I bid every one among you not to think of himself more highly than he ought to think." (Can any of us really plead innocent on that score?) Thinking too highly of ourselves infuses a dark, negative element into the Christian fellowship. It is what separates us from one another, setting the ground for feelings of hurt and rejection, jealousy and resentment. What can we do about it? Well, keeping in mind what we discussed above, the one thing we should certainly *not* do is to hide it (from ourselves and from those who know us best) beneath a surface of false politeness and friendliness. So Paul says, "Let love be *genuine.*" Let it be true. Let it be full.

For love to be full, we must honestly confront the negative feelings we have about one another. Only then can they be rooted out of the heart as well as out of the fellowship. Love becomes genuine as we become genuine. There is no shortcut.

REFLECT | *Our love cannot be genuine and full unless we deal with the negative feelings we have toward one another. What negative feelings do you have toward people you live with, toward your friends, and in the church fellowship? What can you do with these negative feelings?*

Day 7   Inside Out

READ | Matthew 23:1–28

Woe to you, scribes and Pharisees, hypocrites! for you cleanse the outside of the cup and of the plate, but inside they are full of extortion and rapacity. You blind Pharisee! first cleanse the inside of the cup and of the plate, that the outside also may be clean. (vv. 25–26)

Jesus condemns the scribes and Pharisees because of their hypocrisy. The word *hypocrite* comes from a word that originally had to do with acting on a stage, taking on a role, pretending to be someone you are not. In the eyes of Jesus, these men were playing a part, more invested in their outward performances and appearances than in the integrity of their lives. It is important to remember that, as leaders in their faith, they did not set out to be hypocrites. No one says, "My life's ambition is to be hypocritical." But they certainly became hypocrites, as they grew more interested in what showed on the outside, and less interested in what moved around on the inside.

Now, Jesus was not encouraging "bad behavior." But neither was he blinded by "good behavior." He looked behind outward appearances and saw what was in the hearts of his listeners. "For the LORD sees not as man sees; man looks on the outward appearance, but the LORD looks on the heart" (1 Samuel 16:7). And in the hearts of the Pharisees, he saw self-deception and corruption.

Unsettling as this may be, there is a lesson here for every Christian, and especially for the Christian who might say immediately, "Boy, I'm glad I'm not like that!" When we have made a habit of denying our most negative emotions—those ugly, wrong, unacceptable feelings—we have entered the path to hypocrisy. It is not that we want to be hypocrites. But hypocrisy is the inevitable result of lying to ourselves and to others about the ways we really feel. We need a new connection between what is moving around us on the inside and the way we are acting on the outside. It is not our behavior that needs to change, but our hearts.

If what stirs within our hearts is not true, then even the brightest words from our lips and the most pleasant expressions on our faces will carry a certain emptiness. Have you ever been surprised at a friend or a loved-one's hurt reaction to something you said or did—when you intended something good and you tried to *be* good, but somehow it came out all wrong? This may actually be a helpful sign that hypocrisy is at work. This may be time to look at how you are really feeling.

Facing our emotions—all of them, both pleasant and ugly—is the healthiest way to a freer and fuller life. Learning to freely express those feelings that bring lightness and joy, and to face and deal with those feelings that bring darkness and pain, is part of what it means to become a human being, fully alive, fully living to the glory of God.

REFLECT | *During this week, what emotions have you faced within yourself— what pleasant ones, what ugly ones? What do you intend to do about them?*

Week 10 Accepting the Real You

The Plan

EATING RIGHT

- Examine your previous weight goals and revise them if necessary.
- Check your portions this week and see if you can cut down anywhere—a smaller piece of meat, a little less butter or salt, for example.
- Measure your waist and hips this week.

LIVING WELL

- Keep counting your steps!
- Name your blessings and write them in your journal. Add new ones each day. Write three positive things about yourself.

LOVING GOD

- Read a psalm each day this week along with your daily reading. This will only add a minute or two, and it will be a blessing.

THOUGHT **"** Jesus, what didst thou find in me
That thou hast dealt so lovingly!
How great the joy that thou hast brought,
So far exceeding hope or thought!
Jesus my Lord, I thee adore:
O make me love thee more and more. **"**

(Henry Collins, 1827–1919)

W HO AM I? Who do I pretend to be? What's really going on inside me?

I am outgoing, talkative, and spontaneous. I love people, and I love to entertain and throw a wonderful party. However, six years ago when Maggie Davis asked me to write down ten good things about myself, I froze. It was a shock to me that I could not do this. I tried and I tried, and when I went back to her office a week later I told her I could not complete the task she had put before me. I could not put in writing ten good things about myself.

Why could I not do this? Because the real me was not what people saw on the outside. I had for most of my life succeeded in making people think I am confident, capable, and secure. The truth is that I have always had a very low opinion of myself. And if you have a low of opinion of yourself, and a weight struggle, too, this is how you might start thinking: "Why bother?" "What difference does it make, anyway?" "I will never be as thin as she is" or "I will never be as confident as he is."

It was time to take stock of all God had done in my life and own it for myself. And if it meant writing ten good things about myself on a piece of paper to have this healing cemented in my life, then I was going to do it. It took me almost four weeks and much help from Christian friends, but I did it. It was time to stop thinking negative things about myself to protect me. This had been a lifelong bad habit of mine. I had become comfortable with not accepting myself and with believing that I was inferior to others.

Maggie led me in a different direction when in essence she said, "Let's get over those bad things you believe about yourself, and let's start looking for a new you." Yet, I was comfortable with being uncomfortable with myself, and I didn't even know it. Of course there were ten good things I could say about myself. God had been a part of my life for many years. He was living in me and through me.

And so I began the process of writing one thing at a time until I could write ten good things about myself. I know now that this is a problem with many people. When I discuss this experience in a 3D group, I almost always hear a gasp or see an expression of panic come over a face across the table. This is too often the case for anyone who is even slightly overweight. If you identify with my struggle, I challenge you this week to start a list of ten positive things about yourself.

A plaque sits on my desk at home entitled "Top Ten Great Things about Carol." It came from my young friends in the office years ago. The truth has set me free, just as the Bible says it will do. And I pray that the same thing will happen you—through the devotional readings for this week, through prayer, and through sharing with others. My habit pattern of interiorly putting myself down was broken when I wholeheartedly recognized myself as a woman of God with gifts at both home and work: that is the real me. I forget this sometimes, and I have to be reminded, but now I do know who I am, and I know the work God has done in my life.

WHEN YOU PARTICIPATE IN A COVENANTED FELLOWSHIP such as a 3D group for twelve weeks or more, you have an opportunity to let down your guard for perhaps the first time. This is a time when you are free to learn more about yourself. And maybe, like me, you are going to have to move out of the comfortable rut you have lived in. Pray for the vision to see yourself from God's point of view. Ask your friends to help you.

This week's lessons are intended to point you in the direction of the real you. What do you *really* believe? Get rid of the falseness in your life. It's time to stop pretending. In your close friendships and in your group of supporters, you are ready to look in the mirror and be honest with God about who you really are. He already knows you and accepts and loves you, anyway! As you find out who you really are, the changes you want will truly happen. Have faith!

Accepting the Body You Have

Eating right will not necessarily—or by itself—make you a virtuous person, but you may discover your real self in this process. As you have heard several times from Carol and me, there is a profound connection between your mind, your body, and your spirit. What you do for your body is connected to what you do for your mind and your spirit. In all three aspects, there is much more to learn about yourself. Accepting yourself can mean feeling that you have learned from past mistakes. It can be a feeling of having gained from the experiences you have had so far in your journey. And it can bring with it confidence and the expectation that you will do even better in the future.

Many of the images we see in the media are of taller than average models with smaller than average frames who may actually be underweight, anorexic, or bulimic. We also see television and film stars who struggle with the challenges of weight loss and weight maintenance. They may have personal trainers, personal chefs, and plastic surgeons, but they still have to make the choices of what and how much they will eat. Don't let the media images distract you from eating right and living well on your terms.

Accepting the real you includes accepting your body's needs and adapting your diet to where you are in your life. The increased caloric demands and the need to eat more during pregnancy and breastfeeding are adaptations that we all accept. Cutting back once those nutritional demands no longer exist is a challenge that many women can identify with. Decreased caloric needs as you age are subtler and often go unrecognized until a medical problem develops. Your caloric and nutrient needs will change, especially after menopause. Your caloric and nutrient needs will also change as you lose weight, so further assessment and adjustments will need to be made to ensure that your current Calorie level still meets your needs. Be aware that as you lose weight, your body has to do less work now that you are no longer carrying around extra weight.

Understanding Your Size

Take a few minutes this week and reflect on your body size and type and how it relates to your diet. Part of getting to know the right portions for you may be based on how tall you are. This may be a real challenge for women of short stature. Eating with taller individuals who have higher caloric needs, such as your husband or children, can be difficult if your requirements are significantly lower. The typical recommendation of a three-ounce (85-gram) serving of meat the size of a deck of cards may be too large if you are less than five feet (152 centimeters) tall and are post-menopausal. By the same token, it may be too small if you are a man who is six feet three inches (192 centimeters) tall.

Do you know if you have a small, medium, or large frame? If you have been overweight for most of your life, you may assume that you have a large frame, or you may think you have "big bones." You can determine this simply by taking your dominant hand (for example, the right one if you're right-handed) and wrapping your thumb and middle finger around your opposite wrist. If your fingers just meet, you have a medium frame; if they overlap, you have a small frame; if they don't meet, you have a large frame. The size of your body frame may mean that you are meant to weigh more or less than the average person of the same height. This may be a difference of only 5 to 15 pounds (2.25 to 6.8 kilos) in what you should weigh, but knowing your frame size is just one additional piece of self-knowledge that may help you or your healthcare professional determine a good weight for you.

Let's talk briefly again about Body Mass Index and your Body Fat. I mentioned earlier that BMI is a quick way to estimate your Body Fat content using your height and weight. But if a person is very fit and they have a low fat content and a large amount of muscle for their height, they can have a BMI that appears to put them into the next higher weight and risk category. **Women especially may find that their body fat lessens and their muscle mass increases when they increase their**

exercise. This added muscle might mask the actual loss of fat and make you feel that you are not losing fast enough or that you are not seeing the numbers on the scale that you want.

In my office we routinely measure body fat and lean, in order to determine the degree of fitness and health risk for my clients. If you are curious about your actual body fat level at this point, you may want to seek out a healthcare professional or a physical trainer who can perform this quick test for you. And you may want to repeat this two to four times a year as a way of evaluating your progress in maintaining a healthy weight in the future.

If you have made the commitment to your group or to yourself to weigh weekly while following the 3D plan, here's a word of caution: for women of child-bearing age I recommend that you also check your weight right after your menstrual period is over and jot it down on the calendar. Weighing at that time of the month will be a more accurate reflection of your long-term progress and eliminate the daily or weekly fluctuations that can accompany your hormonal cycle.

If you find that you plateau at any point for more than a couple of weeks and you still want to lose more weight, this is the time to reassess. Even though you may be eating well, you may need to reduce the portions again. Alternatively, you could step up your calorie expenditure by 100 to 200 Calories per day for a week. That could mean walking an extra 15 to 30 minutes per day or an additional 2000 to 4000 steps per day.

Are you wearing clothes that fit your body shape now, or are you still buying clothes that are too large or too small? Are you afraid to discard clothes that no longer fit for fear that you will regain weight and need them again? If you don't want to throw out or give away these clothes, we recommend removing them from your day-to-day closet and storing them out of sight. The only clothes in your closet now should be the ones that fit well, that you enjoy wearing, and that you feel good in, even if that is just two or three outfits!

If you have been losing weight, you may also have issues with poor muscle tone and/or excess skin. If this is the case, try to step up your exercise, including strength or resistance as well as cardiovascular exercise. You may want to consider using a video, taking a class, or working with a personal trainer who can help you tone your muscles and target certain areas of your body. You may want to discuss the issue of excess skin with your physician.

Tips for Men

Let's be honest: your pant size is not necessarily the same as your waist measurement. And your waist measurement may be a better indicator than family history of your risk for chronic diseases such as diabetes. As little as a 2-inch (5 cm.) increase in waist size from 34 inches (86 cm.) to 36 inches (91 cm.) doubles your risk for diabetes, and the risk rises with each increase in your waist measurement. So don't be content with 40-inch (101 cm.)-waist slacks even if you've been wearing that size for the last ten years. The abdominal fat above your belt may have increased even if your clothing size hasn't changed. Have someone else measure your waist occasionally as you're making changes. That's the best indicator that you're losing weight and eating right. Aim for 1 inch (2.5 cm.) less for your next goal rather than a specific weight. (Visit www.3DYourWholeLife.com for more information on waist measurement and related health risks.)

Maggie Davis

Week **10** Daily Devotionals

Theme for the Week TRUTH

Verse to Memorize *You will know the truth,*
and the truth will make you free.
—JOHN 8:32

Day 1   The Liberating Power of the Truth

READ | John 8:31–59

If you continue in my word, you are truly my disciples, and you will know the truth, and the truth will make you free. (vv. 31–32)

The eighth chapter of the Gospel of John records a conversation—a debate, really—between Jesus and several religious authorities of his time. At first glance, some of the exchange seems fairly theological and abstract. But Jesus was making a clear point, and his listeners were not getting it.

The first part of the chapter tells the story of a woman caught in adultery. In order to test Jesus' commitment to the righteousness of God, the scribes and Pharisees brought the woman to Jesus for his judgment. "What do you say about her?" they asked, accusatively. You know the rest. Without ever excusing the woman for her actions, Jesus successfully confronted her accusers with their hypocrisy and self-righteousness, pardoned the woman, and sent her on her way with the charge, "Do not sin again" (v. 11).

It was in response to that bold action that the Jewish leaders began to scrutinize Jesus' words and to interrogate him regarding his authority. This was not a friendly audience. Nevertheless, Jesus vigorously engaged in the argument, challenging his listeners to take a hard look at themselves, at the ways in which they were acting, and at the things they were thinking. He pulled no punches. Something vital was seriously amiss, and, at times, he used harsh words to point this out—"You cannot bear to hear my word. You are of your father the devil" (vv. 43–44). Why such strong language? Because Jesus Christ, the Son of God, had perfectly clear insight into something that they could not see—that their arguments were false because their lives were built upon lies!

In these past weeks, we have touched upon the importance of honesty for the sake of becoming whole persons, growing to be better disciples, and uniting more closely with our brothers and sisters in the Lord. This week, we will focus on those things that thwart us from that kind of honesty. We will look more closely at what it means to live in the truth by also looking at the lies we believe that run counter to that truth. Perhaps this is a new thought to you. Most of us were brought up under the clear and commendable instruction that telling lies was and always will be entirely unacceptable behavior. What was probably less an issue, however, was the idea that lies can be not only things that we say but also things that we believe, and therefore live by.

We all form our thinking and prioritize our actions according to the things we believe. Beliefs are like the foundation stones. However, what if some of the things we believe are simply not true in the first place? What misshapen forms exist in a life whose building blocks include lies? Jesus said, "If you continue in my word . . . you will know the truth." Here is a clue to how we come to live in the truth. Jesus Christ not only has the truth, he *is* the Truth, and we can expect his active help as we seek to know more and more of the truth that sets us free.

REFLECT | *Can you think of one "truth" in your life that turned out later to be a lie? How has knowing that changed your life? What makes it difficult to face the lies we believe?*

Day 2   If the Light in You Is Darkness

READ | Matthew 6

But if your eye is not sound, your whole body will be full of darkness. If then the light in you is darkness, how great is the darkness! (v. 23)

The Sermon on the Mount, recorded in Matthew 5–7, is one of the most concentrated collections of all the teachings of Jesus. In these dense chapters we read the life-altering truths of the kingdom of God, in words of comfort—"Blessed are the poor in spirit"; of instruction—"Pray then like this"; of warning—"Beware of practicing your piety before men"; of invitation— "Ask, and it will be given you"; and of explanation—"The eye is the lamp of the body." What does this last statement mean, *The eye is the lamp of the body?* Many of the teachings that surround these two short sentences (vv. 22–23) that concern the eye are direct imperatives: "do this" and "don't do that." So what is this that Jesus is saying about "the eye"?

Remember that Jesus came to present the truths of the kingdom of God to a world that had become blind to the sights and deaf to the sounds of heaven. Quoting from the prophet Isaiah, Jesus said: "For this people's heart has grown dull, and their ears are heavy of hearing, and their eyes they have closed, lest they should perceive with their eyes, and hear with their ears, and understand with their heart, and turn for me to heal them" (Matthew 13:15). In other words, the world is in darkness because its inhabitants can no longer see the light of God.

As the "lamp of the body," the eye is intended, in a spiritual sense, to let in the light, so that the whole person can be filled with divine radiance. But, if the eye is "not sound," then what fills the inner being can be only darkness, for there is only one Source of light, and that is the Light of the world himself.

We all have our "blind spots," those places where it is difficult for us to see things as they really are. For example, it is often the case that we are blind to certain unpleasant truths about those closest to us—our children, our spouse, or our friends. It is almost always the case that we do not see ourselves as we really are. We fixate on certain traits while overlooking others. It may be that what we *want* to see prevents us from seeing what we *should* see; it may be that unhealed hurts, even traumas, have left our vision of life distorted or darkened; it may be that our desire to see what is true is actually weaker than our desire to be right or to be comfortable. Whatever the reasons, we must admit that our eyes are not sound and that we cannot heal them by ourselves. This is why we need the Light that comes *from* God ("I am the light of the world," said Jesus) and that comes *through one another* ("You are the light of the world," said Jesus).

Living in the kingdom of God means, in part, to see things as God sees them, to have his light shed upon even the darkest places in our lives, so that we may be whole. It behooves us, therefore, to have our spiritual vision healed so that we can accurately perceive the things that are true—about God, about the world, and about ourselves. Only then can we be "full of light."

REFLECT | *Ask the Holy Spirit this week to point out just one "blind spot" in your life. What is it? What do you need in order to have it healed? What effect might it have on you to see certain aspects of your life as God sees them?*

Day 3   The Devil's Tempting Lies

READ | Acts 19:1–20

And a number of those who practiced magic arts brought their books together and burned them in the sight of all; and they counted the value of them and found it came to fifty thousand pieces of silver. So the word of the Lord grew and prevailed mightily. (vv. 19–20)

The whole area around Ephesus was shaken and affected by the gospel. God's power was evidenced in the changed lives, the miracles, and the healings, both physical and emotional, that accompanied the preaching of Paul.

Not unexpectedly, the devil sought to frustrate and hinder the work, but God's word prevailed over all opposition. This passage clearly shows the irresistible influence of the truth, as we read the summary of two years' work by Paul and his fellow missionaries in this pagan, Greek city. One of the marvelous fruits of this work is described by Luke: those newly converted to faith in Christ came to the apostles, "confessing and divulging their practices," and, in highly dramatic fashion, casting them from their lives (v. 18). Through his servants, God had put the power of divine truth alongside the power of the enemy's lies—lies by which these people had lived—and the truth had prevailed. The result was the birth of a new community of faith, a new group of liberated people. The lies that had once bound them to ways of evil had been soundly defeated through the bold arguments and pleadings of Paul about the kingdom of God (v. 8).

The delusions by which Satan seeks to bind us are based on our all-too-human, but sinful, desire to be God. (Remember the snake's enticement to Eve?—"You will be like God," Genesis 3:5). His, of course, is the same nature, to the nth degree. The Bible tells us that the insatiable ambition to take God's place was the cause of the devil's own downfall. He recognizes something familiar in fallen human nature, and appeals to it with his lies. He offers (but cannot deliver) power and praise, instant gratification, pleasure without pain, authority without responsibility, and success without cost. (Take a look at the temptations he set before Jesus, Matthew 4:1–11.) Such things naturally appeal to our desire for ease, to our sense of vanity and entitlement, to our fears and anxieties. As long as we live and breathe on this earth, these things will hold for us a certain allure. But make no mistake. They are nothing but counterfeits and shadows—because they are lies.

The new Christians of Ephesus made a costly down payment upon their intention to be disciples of Jesus Christ. They brought all their manuals of sorcery and magic, signs of their deep commitment to the lies they had been living to that point, and burned them in the sight of everyone. The value represented an investment that is staggering to the imagination, even by today's standards. It was a price that they were happy to pay, for the truth had brought them a new freedom that was worth every penny, and more.

REFLECT | *What aspects of the devil's lies hold the most temptation for you? A way to think about this might be to read the story of Jesus' temptation in the wilderness. Which of those temptations would have been hardest for you to resist? Why?*

Day 4 How Long Will You Seek After Lies

READ | Psalms 4–5

O men, how long shall my honor suffer shame? How long will you love vain words, and seek after lies? (4:2)

Second Samuel 15 records the jealous betrayal of David by his son, Absalom. Coveting the throne of Israel for himself, Absalom schemed to steal it from his father, not so much by force as by stealth. To his eventual destruction (see 2 Samuel 18:6–15), he succeeded. He and his treasonous co-conspirators lied their way into the hearts of the people, gained their support, and came to occupy the city of Jerusalem. King David, and those faithful to him, were forced to steal away in the night. The writer tells us that, as they fled, they wept (2 Samuel 15:30).

It was under these dire circumstances—betrayed by his own son, abandoned by his own people, and exiled from his beloved city—that David turns to the Lord and writes these two psalms of prayer. They contain the sounds, both of his desperate petition to God for help and deliverance—"Hearken to the sound of my cry, my King and my God" (5:2)—and of his confidence that those who have deceived him will ultimately come to ruin—"Thou destroyest those who speak lies" (5:6).

Speaking prophetically for God, David directly addresses his betrayers in 4:2 as, "O men." But David deliberately chooses a Hebrew word that means far more than gender. It is a word denoting distinction and honor, a sarcastic way of saying that these "big shots" are really just little men, demeaned and discredited by their own duplicity. It is the irony of God to give these men a title of honor that has no substance, for it refers only to their own high opinion of themselves.

Upon what is this opinion based? Nothing but utter lies: "How long will you seek after lies?"; "There is no truth in their mouth"; "They flatter with their tongue." These were not honorable men, just boastful bullies. Absalom promised his followers a quick and easy way to prestige and power. His entire plan was based upon lies and deceptions—that he had a right to the throne, that the people would love him if he held position and power, that those who followed him would dwell secure in their newfound (stolen) status. Flattery and delusion spread through Absalom's camp like a plague, dooming it to inevitable destruction.

The example of Absalom may be extreme, but it contains an explicit lesson for the Christian: departure from the truth always leads to ruin. A course that begins with false self-justifications (I could be a better king than he is!), and deceptively reasonable claims (why shouldn't I have whatever I want?), will eventually lead to outright rebellion against God. David's prayers remind us that God will not tolerate lies forever, that faithfulness will ultimately have its reward, and that truthfulness is a powerful expression of trust in the Lord.

REFLECT | *Think about the things that you really want out of life. What lies might you be tempted to live by (indeed, what lies do you live by) in order to pursue those desires? How can the words of David's prayers be helpful to you?*

Day 5　Misplaced Trust

READ | Jeremiah 7:1–20

Behold, you trust in deceptive words to no avail. (v. 8)

The people of Judah believed that since they had the temple in their midst—meaning that God had favored them by choosing their city as his dwelling place—they would always know peace and prosperity, regardless of the way they actually lived. This deceptive self-assurance was drummed into them. Rest easy, they thought, for here is "the temple of the LORD, the temple of the LORD, the temple of the LORD" (v. 4).

The prophet Jeremiah warns them that trusting in such a misleading message ("deceptive words"), while all the time living unfaithfully to his precepts, will only lead to their demise. Go to Shiloh,

he challenges them. If you think that God will not punish wickedness, even in the most sacred of places, see what is left of that chosen city, once so wealthy and powerful (vv. 12–14). God holds the people accountable for their actions. Their confidence in lying words is severely misplaced. They come to the temple saying that their trust is in the Lord, while all the while they live their daily lives going after other gods. Their actions speak loudest of all about where they truly put their trust.

Yesterday we explored the betrayal of Absalom, who deceived others (as well as himself) by beguiling them into trusting his methods. On the other hand, David's commitment to truth and integrity, even when under duress, was actually an expression of his trust in the Lord. Today's is a similar story. Our trust will betray us if it is misplaced. Things that are not true will not save us. They *cannot* save us. We dare not build our lives upon such flimsy foundations.

Instead, God offers truth to be the enduring building blocks of our faith. We know the folly of some of the delusions we have entertained. There are still more for all of us to see. Rest assured that, out of his great love for us, God will lead us to discover and to discard each one of them.

Here are some common "deceptive words":
—Peace at any price is good.
—I must do anything I can to avoid having my feelings hurt, or hurting the feelings of others.
—If you love me, you will accept me and let me be just as I am.
What is untrue about each of these beliefs? What would be the truth that counters each of these lies?

When you discover a "deceptive word" in which you have placed your trust, try praying something like this: "Lord, I confess to you that I have believed this lie: (name what it is). I take responsibility for believing this, and I am sorry. I accept your forgiveness. In your name, I renounce this lie and all its effects in my life. Before you, I state this truth: (name the thing that is true, in opposition to the lie). I ask you to fill my heart with this truth, and let it bear fruit in my life. In the name of Jesus, I pray. Amen."

Day 6   Obeying the Truth

READ | Galatians 5:1–25

You were running well; who hindered you from obeying the truth? (v. 7)

The Christians of Galatia were young in their faith. As such, they were not yet stable and mature. They had heard Paul's preaching about salvation in Jesus Christ. They had welcomed the message, professed their faith, and received the gift of the Holy Spirit into their lives. Now, having come to know God (4:9), they had set forth upon a new way of life in the power of the Spirit.

It wasn't long, however, before the Galatians wandered from their newfound course. Others, coming after Paul, told them that, in addition to believing in Jesus, they also had to be circumcised and adhere in all respects to the Jewish law. The message seemed convincing, and the Galatians were persuaded that they would become superior Christians if they followed this new plan. Paul was furious with those who had come and unsettled these converts. He had repeatedly risked his life in order to bring the Good News to this region. Now, these deceptive "Judaizers" had slipped in behind him, sowing

confusion and controversy in the church. Paul feared that the infant body of believers would turn away from the truth and follow the ways of "a different gospel" (1:6).

The Letter to the Galatians could therefore be called a word of "correction," in which the apostle is admonishing his readers for their "foolishness" and calling them back to the truth. "You were running well," he says; "who hindered you from obeying the truth?" We know *who* hindered them. The real question is: what made the false message they heard so appealing to them? Probably one of the same things that appeal to all of us—it held out the promise that they could be better than anyone else. "They make much of you, but for no good purpose," Paul protested (4:17). Rather than remaining utterly dependent upon the undeserved grace of God, the Galatians succumbed to the temptation to "be right."

In many respects, the desire to be right is one of the Christian's deadliest foes, because it is a counterfeit for being obedient. Rightness, as the soul's objective, has about it a subtle, (though nevertheless destructive) pride that robs God of his glory and nourishes our self-righteous, high opinion of ourselves. As our own sense of "rightness" increases, our dependence upon God's "righteousness" decreases. Before we know it, warns Paul, we have come to depend upon ourselves—upon our own good deeds and good motives— to be our salvation.

This is one of the most difficult and most important lessons we have to learn. "Walking by the Spirit" keeps us in a state of humility before God and one another, because it prevents us from boasting "in the flesh," that is, in ourselves. But it is easier said than done: we must spend our entire Christian lives in learning how to live this way. Once you have set upon this course, do not be surprised if God sends a "letter" to you now and then, correcting you for your pride, and calling you back to obey the truth.

REFLECT | *In what subtle (or not so subtle) ways do you depend upon your own sense of rightness in order to be at peace? What areas of secret pride do you hold in your heart that make you feel more acceptable to yourself, to others, and to God?*

Day 7   I Would Have Been Untrue

READ | Psalm 73

If I had said, "I will speak thus," I would have been untrue to the generation of thy children. (v. 15)

One thing can always be said about the psalms: they are honest! Here we find the psalmist freely admitting that there is a whole list of things he believes that are untrue. And in his darkest times, when his feet stumble and his soul is embittered, that is precisely when these untrue things rise to the surface. (Some true things arise, as well, but more about that later.)

In his time of trouble, the psalmist looks about him, and can see only the prosperity of the wicked (v. 3). These people appear healthier, less disturbed, and more successful than those who strive to do right. They grow wealthier each day, enjoying ease of life and peace of mind. Their pride and their arrogance are obvious—"their eyes swell out with fatness, their hearts overflow with follies"—as they live in constant contempt of others, even looking down disdainfully upon heaven itself. Worst of all—adding insult to his own injured soul—the psalmist hears them being praised by others, as if they had no faults at all! He, on the other hand, grows despondent with his maladies. His misfortunes make him hopeless and bitter. "It's no use trying to serve God and keep one's hands innocent of wrong," he despairs. "It is all for naught."

But wait. The psalmist cannot let his complaint go unchallenged. He cannot let these words, as honest as they are, stand as the final truth. *If I had said, "I will speak thus," I would have been untrue to the generation of thy children.* In his plight, he goes into God's house, and there he discovers something more, something deeper, something "more true" than the way he was seeing things (vv. 16–20).

God is not fooled by the appearance of the wicked, nor unmindful of the psalmist's need. In the end, both will receive their reward from the just hand of the Almighty. The psalmist knows that this is the truth that prevails over all other passing images. God is *good.* To give any lesser word the last say would be a betrayal of his own soul, as well as the souls of others.

We all harbor certain lies and "half-truths" in our own hearts, and not until times of trial do they usually show their ugly heads. Bitterness makes us "stupid and ignorant," as the psalmist put it. It is a menace to others as well as to ourselves. When we live as if the accusations we hold against God are the final reality, we cripple our own faith and we cause others to stumble. Take heart from the psalmist, however. Once he honestly makes his complaint before God, he lets God correct his incomplete vision of things. Then, he can be true to his listeners and say of the Lord, "I have made the Lord GOD my refuge, that I may tell of *all* thy works."

REFLECT | *What "half-truths" do you know you believe about God? What "whole-truths" do you need to declare in order to be true to God, to yourself, and to others?*

Week 11 The Battle for Your Mind

The Plan

EATING RIGHT

▓ Plan your dinner menu every night this week. Then do your grocery list, being aware of what you have learned.

▓ Write in your journal any food changes you are making.

LIVING WELL

▓ Add another 200 steps to your daily total. For fun, try walking to a destination, such as your favorite store or coffee-shop.

▓ Be aware of your thoughts throughout the day. What is your first thought in the morning? Are you putting yourself down, or building yourself up? Do you berate yourself about some aspect of your body? This week, choose to battle negative thoughts with positive ones.

▓ Go for a walk with a friend or a neighbor this week. Add your walking partner to your prayer list.

LOVING GOD

▓ This week, take Sunday and completely "unplug" yourself from the usual rush of life. Turn off your computer, cell phone, and PDA, and ignore the unpaid bills or the deck that needs painting. Ask God to guide you through this day of rest.

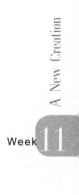

A New Creation

Week 11

The Battle for Your Mind

Y OUR MIND IS A BATTLEGROUND. From the moment you wake up in the morning until the moment you go to sleep at night, a battle is going on. How many times have you asked yourself, "Where did that thought come from?"

Pause for a minute and recall what the first thought was that entered your mind this morning. Was it a good thought, or not?

I realized long ago that I could set the direction of my life by realizing and changing the first thoughts that come into my life in the morning: "Oh, I have so much to do today that I dread getting up"; "I hate the thought of going to that meeting this morning"; "I wish it was Friday"; "I am so behind in everything that I don't want to even get up."

When I start my day this way, the tone is set; I am off to a negative start. It is not hard to think of where I will be by 10:00 AM—probably eating a donut at the office!

Let's consider new thoughts for the new day: Thank you, God, that there have been no family emergencies in the night; Thank you, Lord, that I am alive, and so is my husband; Thank you, Lord, that I have good health and that I can walk and see this morning.

Sometimes I say a prayer that I taught my children years ago: "Good morning, God. This is your day. I am your child. Show me the way." This is a simple prayer, but it is a profound way to start a new day.

A wonderful teaching on this subject
is available at www.3DYourWholeLife.com
Order it today. It was this tape called
"The Battle for Your Mind" that opened my heart to
understanding the battle that I was in daily with my mind.

All sorts of thoughts invade our minds. We need to do battle against the evil thoughts that invade our minds at the conscious level. As we seek to do battle with our conscious thoughts, the Holy Spirit will do battle for us against any evil thoughts buried at the unconscious level.

> The good news is that, by faith and with God's help, this battle can be won—daily.

The good news is that, by faith and with God's help, this battle can be won—daily. Try this week to capture your first thought in the morning. Make a conscious effort to focus only on those things that encourage you to live well. Make a decision to battle all negativity and bad thoughts. You will arm yourself with faith and walk into this day believing that those thoughts can indeed be taken captive under Christ. By his grace, they will.

THOUGHT   **❝ Daughter of Jerusalem, go ahead and walk with a joyful heart in the way of contemplation of the Lord.**
Run the course well. Run it loving.
Run it purely.
Run it with discretion and humility. ❞

(Elisabeth of Schonau, 1129-1165)

Evaluate Labels

I recently examined a loaf of whole grain bread in my grocery store. I looked at the list of ingredients and was happy to see that sugar was absent, fiber was 3 grams per slice, and the bread contained whole wheat and whole grain rye as well as sesame seeds, poppy seeds, and pumpkin seeds. Then I checked the serving size that was used as a base for the Nutrition Facts: 1 slice of bread. There were 20 servings in the package, or so the label read. I counted the slices myself and there were 15. Some slices were as large as 2 regular slices of bread, and the slices at the end of the loaf were tiny. No wonder it's confusing to buy and eat well!

We must rely on our own hunger and satisfaction to determine a serving that is appropriate for us. And this means trying to eat less than we did previously if we want our body to change. Eating right implies eating proactively. It means keeping up on current food and nutrition information, which is constantly being updated. New and valid information may need to be incorporated into your food life. It may also mean:

■ Comparing food labels, nutrition facts, and ingredient lists;

■ Evaluating new food products and marketing claims, and not just falling for the hype;

■ Using recipes, cookbooks, magazines, and websites as sources of recipes and seasonal inspiration.

All of this doesn't just start at the grocery store. Do you devote the time that planning a grocery list and shopping deserve? Or do you run into the market for the makings for dinner at 6:00 PM? Do you leave the house without breakfast because you don't have anything quick and convenient to eat? If so, you leave yourself at risk for impulsive, limited, and high-Calorie food choices.

When you eat away from home, do you think about what you will eat before you arrive at a restaurant? Have you checked nutritional information listed on a restaurant's website? Have you called ahead to see what's on the menu and find out if it's possible to get what you want or need if you have a medical diet concern? And most important, have you thought about what you would like to eat, before you are told about the tempting specials that are on the menu tonight?

I was in Portugal about 15 years ago when I became aware of the temptation of the breadbasket in a restaurant. On our first night there my husband and walked to a small local restaurant and were seated for dinner. Just as in our country, a basket of bread was brought to the table before we ordered. They also brought a small piece of the local cheese and some olives. We sampled the bread and took a taste of cheese and olives, all in the name of researching the local foods. We ordered a beautiful fish dinner that we enjoyed thoroughly. When the check came, we found that we had been charged for the order of bread as well as the cheese and the olives. Every meal after that during our trip we became more conscious of making a decision regarding whether or not we were hungry enough to have the bread. I quickly learned to say "no bread, please" in Portuguese.

The road to eating right is filled with billboards, media messages, and misleading food labels that may tempt you to go off track in your selection of foods to eat. You may realize on some level that you are being persuaded to believe what you want to believe about a particular food. You may be in total denial and not even look at the back of the package for the nutrition facts or the list of ingredients.

If you do look at the package, do you know that the portion size on a packaged food is determined by the manufacturer, not by a government agency such as the USDA or the FDA, or by a healthcare professional, such as a nutritionist, a dietitian, or a physician? These portion sizes do not necessarily match classic portions such as the American Dietetic Association Food Exchanges or Dietary Guidelines for Americans or the Food Pyramid. They may be larger or smaller than the portion you actually eat. A particular food may be marketed and labeled with a larger portion to make it appear to be higher in fiber or protein, but that also makes it higher in Calories. That portion may not be the right one for you. There are many processed foods that are marketed with smaller portions than most individuals would eat.

Let's Talk Supplements

The very word *supplement* indicates that these nutrient doses are additions or complements to our usual food intake. They are not meant to be a substitute for consuming a variety of healthy foods. They can be particularly useful if an individual is reducing portions, since eating a smaller volume of food may mean consuming fewer nutrients. They may also be necessary if your needs for a particular nutrient are higher than usual, or if your body has difficulty absorbing a nutrient.

If you do decide to take a multinutrient (multivitamin plus minerals), we recommend selecting one that does not exceed 100% of your daily needs unless you consult your healthcare provider. Excess vitamin intake has been implicated in the progression of conditions such as certain kinds of cancer. But extra supplementation is often necessary to obtain enough calcium, Vitamin D, or other nutrients, especially if you are trying to reduce the amount of food you are eating. The less you eat and the older you get, the more nutritional value you need to get out of every bite—and the more you may need supplementation for certain nutrients. Furthermore, with age you may have a reduced ability to absorb some nutrients, so you may need additional help to consume adequate portions to maintain your health.

Be sure to check with your healthcare provider before taking supplements other than a multivitamin if you are taking prescription medications, since some over-the-counter supplements and herbs may interfere with the action of your prescription.

Maggie Davis

Week **11** Daily Devotionals

Theme for the Week YOUR MIND

Verse to Memorize *We destroy arguments and*
every proud obstacle
to the knowledge of God,
and take every thought captive
to obey Christ.

—2 CORINTHIANS 10:5

Day 1　We Destroy Arguments

READ ｜ 2 Corinthians 10

We destroy arguments and every proud obstacle to the knowledge of God, and take every thought captive to obey Christ. (v. 5)

This week we introduce a subject of both great import and great practicality. Take a moment to think (there's the word already!) about how much of your day is spent using your mind. We are not talking about those innumerable involuntary signals your brain sends to make your body do what it needs to do. We are talking about all the thoughts that fly through your day like grains of sand in a windstorm: "How am I going to get to this?" "What did she mean by that?" "What's going on here?" "I wish I could have that." "Who does he think he is?" "What's next?" "I wish I hadn't said that." "Late again—what will they think?" And on . . . and on . . . and on. . . . There's no stopping these thoughts. Or is there?

Let's face it: the mind is our own personal combat zone. We work out all sorts of problems on that field and, frankly, we create just as many. But, as Christians, we should not believe that ours are the only forces contending upon its ground.

A spiritual battle rages in every child of God—a battle between light and darkness, between the God of truth and the father of lies, between Spirit and the flesh. And the mind is the primary battleground on which the Christian's warfare is fought.

Paul is addressing a particularly arrogant and disobedient group of Christians when he writes to the church in Corinth. Their behavior is misguided, even unholy, because their thoughts are unruly. We are not talking here about massive theoretical ideas and grand philosophies. The minds of these Christians, says Paul, have become captivated by false "arguments" that have grown from passing thoughts into strongholds of misinformation, "proud obstacles" to the will of God.

This is where things get practical. Go back to that endless list of thoughts that scurry through your mind all day. Which ones keep repeating themselves? Which ones fortify your own sense of "rightness," or someone else's "wrongness?" Which ones tempt you to act in ways that you know are counter to the will of God? Which ones bring ideas and images that demean others or distort your vision of God? Which ones can you no longer "get out of your head"? These are the thoughts that constitute "arguments and proud obstacles to the knowledge of God," building blocks for the enemy's strongholds in our souls. They are a force to contend with, and the only countermeasure strong enough to destroy them—or, better yet, to prevent their assault in the first place—is to take every one of them "captive to obey Christ."

REFLECT | *Answer the questions in the above paragraph as honestly as you can. Choose one of those thoughts that you know harasses your mind. What truth can you wield, as your own weapon, in order to capture that thought and make it obedient to Christ?*

THOUGHT 66 Every minute you are thinking of evil, you might have been thinking of good instead. Refuse to pander to a morbid interest in your own misdeeds. Pick yourself up, be sorry, shake yourself, and go on again. 99

(Evelyn Underhill, 1875-1941)

Day 2 What Can We Learn From Judas?

READ | Luke 22:1–33

Then Satan entered into Judas called Iscariot, who was of the number of the twelve; he went away and conferred with the chief priests and captains how he might betray him to them. (vv. 3–4)

Where did Judas go wrong? There is nothing in the Gospels to indicate that his mind and heart were already corrupted when he began his life as a disciple of Jesus. Surely he did not join this sacred company with the idea that he would someday become a traitor to his Master. What then happened, through the intervening years, that led Judas to abandon his initial intention to follow Jesus and to finally make such a heinous decision to betray him?

In the Gospel accounts there are clues of a possible answer to this mystery. For example, John writes of Judas that, "he was a thief, and as he had the money box he used to take what was put into it" (John 12:6b). Judas was apparently the company treasurer (did you ever wonder how, very practically, Jesus and his disciples lived from day to day?). In that capacity, he had regular responsibility for and access to the funds made available to the group. You can almost picture what happened, can't you? On some occasion, Judas desired a little extra for himself, for something he wanted, or perhaps even needed. What could it hurt to take a coin or two from the box? He may even have told himself that he would try to pay it back but, if he didn't, who would miss it? The next time the opportunity presented itself, the act was easier. And the stealing kept getting easier, and grew more appealing, until the dark day when Judas was offered thirty whole pieces of silver in return for a simple kiss. At that point, his answer was wholly predictable.

What does this suggest? The writer of the Song of Solomon wisely observes that it is the "little foxes" that spoil the vineyard (2:15). The full-on, frontal assaults against our convictions and against the values we hold dear as disciples of Christ—these are easy to recognize for what they are. They are too big to go unnoticed and, therefore, too obvious to go unchallenged. There is no evidence telling us that Judas ever tried to rob the treasury of the Temple! But the little ideas, the vague tempting thoughts, the "harmless" rationalizations we make in our minds, these we fall for many, many times. Eventually, when we have ignored or surrendered to enough of these clandestine temptations, we are ready to be hit by the big one. And no one can be surprised by the sad outcome.

Among other things, the heartbreaking conclusion to Judas' story tells us that the spiritual skirmishes we wage in our minds may actually be more important than the great wars. Spiritual warfare can be subtle as well as severe. Are all those little thoughts that pass through our minds really as innocent and powerless as we would like to think? Apparently not. Before we determine that Judas is altogether different from ourselves, it would be wise for us to consider how he came to his tragic end. Betrayal happens step by tiny step, and many of those steps are taken on the battlefield of the mind.

REFLECT | *What seemingly innocent thoughts or rationalizations have you entertained this week? If they were to have their way, where would (did) they lead you? Or, put another way—what "little foxes" do you recognize prowling around your mind? What will you do about them?*

Day 3   Out of the Abundance of the Heart

READ | Luke 6:17–49

The good man out of the good treasure of his heart produces good, and the evil man out of his evil treasure produces evil; for out of the abundance of the heart his mouth speaks. (v. 45)

The Bible's understanding of the "heart" has to do with the essence of a person's interior being, including the mind. Here lies the center of our identity, the "core of our being," so to speak. This is where the human person "lives" before he or she "acts." This is what

Jesus is saying. The will decides, the eyes look, the hands grasp, and the mouth speaks—and all these actions are motivated and energized by what goes on beneath the surface.

Of course, many of those motivations take place in our subconscious, and we do not even understand what we are doing. Remember back to Week 3, when we referred to Paul's description of this dilemma?—"I do not do the good I want, but the evil I do not want is what I do" (Romans 7:19). Jesus' words give some indication as to why this frustrating condition is true for us all. Deep within our souls, he says, lurk those seminal ideas and motives that will eventually give birth to our words and actions. And, usually, the first place they will make their presence known is in our minds. Then, the next place is often on our lips.

Have you ever surprised yourself (and those around you) when, intending to say something funny, you instead blurted out something that was hurtful or judgmental? Before you knew it, the words were out your mouth. Your attempt to tease turned into a genuine insult, or your innocent explanation took on a clear tone of malicious accusation.

If so, Jesus explains the reason. Somewhere, within your own heart and mind, "evil treasure" is being stored in the form of buried anger, unforgiven hurt, pent-up judgment, or lingering resentment. Whatever the spiritual currency, it will finance the payout.

Someone has said that a harmless thought turns into a dangerous temptation the minute we begin to converse with it. (Just recall what happened when Eve began to answer the questions put to her by the snake.) It is inevitable that some of those "conversations" will make their way out in public. This is when we start speaking, albeit unintentionally, the ungodly things that we are really thinking. Yes, part of the remedy is to apologize for the remarks and to be sincerely sorry for the pain they cause. But, unless all we really want is to get over the embarrassment of the moment (which, by the way, is entirely different from conviction of sin), we will set out to discover their source.

Why did I say such a thing? This is a question to ponder in your own heart, to prayerfully bring before the Holy Spirit (the Spirit of truth) and, if you are humble enough to listen, to bring to a friend. There *is* an answer to the question, and chances are quite good that, while you may not like it, you will most surely want to do something about it.

REFLECT │ *Beyond "Why did I say such a thing?" an important question is, "Why am I thinking such a thing?" What words have you used this week, or what thoughts have you entertained, that require this kind of examination?*

Day 4　Blinded Minds

READ │ 2 Corinthians 4

In their case the god of this world has blinded the minds of the unbelievers, to keep them from seeing the light of the gospel of the glory of Christ, who is the likeness of God. (v. 4)

We have said that the mind is the prime ground upon which the forces of "light" and "darkness" wage war (tomorrow we will have more to say about the spiritual character of this battle). Writing to the Christians in Thessalonica, the apostle says: "For you are all sons of light and sons of the day; we are not of the night or of darkness" (1 Thessalonians 5:5). This is a good image to consider when we read the words "the god of this world has *blinded* the minds." By "the god of this world," of course, Paul means the devil, together with his allies. For now, the darkness of his dominion overshadows the world and has successfully blinded some from "seeing" the truth of the Gospel.

Earlier in his letter, Paul wrote of minds that were "hardened" to the brightness of God (3:14). Even as such people could physically read the Scriptures, their eyes remained veiled from perceiving the truth of its message. There is a relationship between the "hardening" and the "blindness" of which Paul speaks. By repeatedly resisting the truth of God—denying those things we don't want to believe, ignoring those corrective words that make us uncomfortable, defending ourselves against every unwelcome admonition—we eventually harden our minds to the convicting power of that truth.

The situation can become quite desperate. When we harden ourselves to the truth of God, our minds become progressively darkened. The self-defensive walls that we build, in order to shield ourselves from the heat, block out the light as well. Eventually, we can no longer discern truth from falsehood, and we grow uncertain about everything except our own rightness in the matter. There is no great mystery here. This is the simple process by which the mind, hardened against seeing its own wrongness, grows more and more unreachable, until it becomes completely "blind."

An extreme example may illustrate the dangers. In his study of some of the spiritual issues behind certain psychological conditions, Rev. Earl Jabay, a clinically trained chaplain, wrote in *The Kingdom of Self*: "This happened in the case of Tom, a splendid young man in his early twenties. Tom had tried for days to argue with me on the hate-filled issues of neo-Nazism, anti-Semitism, and white racism. Finally I turned to Tom and asked, 'Which do you want—to be right on these issues or to get well so you can leave this hospital!' Without a moment's hesitation he answered, 'Be right! I don't care if I never get out of this hospital!'"[4]

If wholeness is God's intention for us (and it most certainly is!), then hardening our minds to the truths God is sending us is a sure way to thwart his plans and prevent our own healing. It is worth considering all those arguments that are going on in our minds. The ones we think we are winning?—we may, in fact, be losing.

REFLECT | *In what areas of your life do you know you are resisting God? Against what uncomfortable truth about yourself do you work most hard to defend yourself? Why?*

Day 5   The Wiles of the Devil

READ | Ephesians 6

Put on the whole armor of God, that you may be able to stand against the wiles of the devil. (v. 11)

According to the dictionary, a "wile" is "a trick or stratagem intended to ensnare or deceive." It is certainly possible for Christians to become too "devil-conscious," and to give unhealthy attention to what we think are evidences of his presence or power. But it is equally possible, and perilous, to disregard his "wiles," or to think that talk about Satan and his methods is simply old-fashioned or irrational. (C.S. Lewis said that convincing the world that Satan does not exist is the devil's greatest, and most successful, lie!) Ignorance of his deceptions is the surest way to be ensnared by them. It is difficult to avoid a trap that you do not see, or, better yet, that you do not believe is set in the first place.

The apostle Paul is exhorting his readers to recognize that there are spiritual enemies arrayed against us. "We are not contending against flesh and blood, but against the principalities, against the powers, against the world rulers of this present darkness, against the spiritual hosts of wickedness in the heavenly places" (v. 12). These are the unseen and evil forces that are at work against us, because they have been at work against God for eons. As God's sons and daughters, we have been enlisted in this fight. If we do not know our enemy's tactics we are sure to fall under his influence.

What are some of the signs that might tell us that the devil's wiles are at work on us? Here are some: when we cannot bear to be criticized or to admit our own failures; when we find ourselves suspicious of someone's motives and we actually look for reasons to feel hurt by them; when we subtly place ourselves into situations where we will be praised for our good deeds; when we begin to think that our situation is hopeless, and even that *we* are hopeless; when we cannot get out of our minds the "awful thing" someone said to us; when we cannot figure out how to make someone like us; when we think that our decision to do something or not do something won't make any difference anyway.

Perhaps there are some other "wiles" with which you are more familiar, because you encounter them more often. In any case, the question is not whether or not the devil will use them against us—the question is, will we do something to fend them off? The mind is the usual battleground in which these tricks must be countered. If, with our minds, we entertain the devil's lies, as if they had merit, then we most surely lay open our hearts to the sting of his fiery darts. The *whole* armor of God is needed to stand against his attacks.

REFLECT | *How should we try to fight against our mind wandering, and encourage spiritually healthy thoughts?*

Day 6   The Renewal of Your Minds

READ | Romans 12

Do not be conformed to this world but be transformed by the renewal of your mind, that you may prove what is the will of God, what is good and acceptable and perfect. (v. 2)

John Greenleaf Whittier (1807–1892) wrote this prayerful hymn:
> Dear Lord and Father of mankind,
> Forgive our foolish ways.
> Reclothe us in our rightful mind,
> In purer lives thy service find,
> In deeper reverence, praise.

"Reclothe our minds," or, in the apostle Paul's words, "renew" them. One of the bitter fruits of the disobedience of our first parents, Adam and Eve, has been the darkening of the human mind that, in turn, has led to all manner of defective thinking and deceitful living. This is why the promise of redemption came through the prophet Isaiah in these timeless words: "The people who walked in darkness have seen a great light; those who dwelt in a land of deep darkness, on them has light shined" (9:2). That light is Jesus Christ, who, shining in our hearts by the power of the Holy Spirit, brings us out of everlasting night!

Isn't it interesting that Paul connects the transformation of our lives with the renewal—one might say, the "enlightening"—of our minds? One commentator on these verses puts it thus: "The children of light, being risen with Christ, have a life of their own—the life of pardoned and reconciled believers: renewed in the spirit of their mind, they breathe a new air, they have new interests and affections, and their sympathies are all heavenly and spiritual."[5] It is no wonder that one of the names for baptism in the early church was "illumination."

However, renewed minds are more than the *result* of our conversion. Paul says that our lives are transformed *by* the renewal of our minds. Our sanctification—our being re-created in the likeness of Christ—is inherently connected to the changing of our minds. Living differently depends upon our thinking differently. And this is a process that takes both time and effort. Yes, the Holy Spirit is the chief "instrument" of our transformation. Without the Breath of God we have no hope of spiritual resuscitation. But he works with the clay that he is given. It is up to us to make every effort in order to present him with our whole selves—body, heart, and mind—so that no part of our lives will remain conformed to the world's image, and all will be renewed into the image of God.

REFLECT | *What are some of the "old" thoughts that you bring with you, from the world, into your Christian life? How do these old thoughts stifle your spiritual growth? With what new thoughts must they be replaced?*

Day 7   The Mind of Christ

READ | 1 Corinthians 2

So also no one comprehends the thoughts of God except the Spirit of God.
(v. 11)

We concluded yesterday's discussion by talking about our lives being transformed—re-created—in the image of God. This is the work of the Holy Spirit, operating together with our own best efforts to yield our whole lives completely into his hands. Paul is particularly concerned that one aspect of that work should take place in the lives of the Corinthian Christians. He is writing to a church that has suffered greatly from internal strife and division. The underlying cause of much of their troubles is that they do not understand God's ways. They think, for example, that a God who is all-powerful and all-wise must therefore value lofty stature and superior intelligence. On the contrary, corrects Paul, God chose what is foolish in the world, what is weak and low and despised, in order to bring about his purposes (1:27–28). Paul says that what they have been thinking about God and about one another is utterly wrong!

In chapter 2, Paul expresses his deep wish that these young Christians could understand a different way. However, he admits, they can never understand God's ways without his Spirit. It is a useless endeavor for the mind of man to grasp the thoughts of God. Therefore, it is part of the transforming work of the Holy Spirit to teach us to think as God thinks. What a mysterious idea. And, it gets even more startling when we read Paul's concluding words to this chapter—*we have the mind of Christ.*

Learning to think the thoughts of God: This sounds grandiose, but it is really quite down-to-earth. If we were made in God's image—that is, to reflect the nature of God with every part of our being—then does it not make sense that our minds, too, were created to think after the thoughts of God? When Paul talks about the "spiritual man," he is not talking about some few, specially endowed people who are head and shoulders above the rest of us. He is talking about you and me—all who "call on the name of our Lord Jesus Christ" (1:2) and who have "received ... the Spirit which is from God" (2:12). The Holy Spirit, dwelling within us, teaches us the mind of our Lord.

Much of this week has been spent discussing the "battle" that goes on in our minds. Today's Scripture reading tells us why that is so. God's thoughts—his priorities and methods, his concerns and ways—are not our thoughts (see Isaiah 55:8–9). Just consider, for example, how much of your day is spent thinking about yourself and how much of it is spent thinking about others; whom do you think God "thinks" about all day? In and of ourselves, we have no hope of having our minds changed. *But*, says Paul, "we have the mind of Christ." No wonder the mind is such a battleground.

REFLECT | *From your reading and your experience this week, what areas of your thinking would you identify as your chief battles? Where does your thinking most need to be changed? In what one new way would you most like to think differently?*

The Plan

EATING RIGHT

Here are **10 strategies** to help you eat right
for **Your Whole Life:**

- Eat early and often.
- Plan meals, purchase ingredients, and prepare for the meal in advance.
- Make real, whole food the core of your meals and snacks.
- Always make changes gradually to let your body, mind, and spirit adjust.
- Avoid trigger foods that make you hungry or cause you to keep eating.
- Be conscious of your automatic eating habits.
- Listen to your hunger and satisfaction signals.
- Be mindful of your portions; eat less each year.
- Eat seasonally and locally whenever possible.
- Include exercise as part of your healthy eating plan.

LIVING WELL

- Exercise is a key ingredient for the 3D plan. Are you ready to add one more day or 500 more steps? Keep counting and keep moving!
- Make a home organization plan, and establish goals for the next twelve weeks. Is there a room that needs an upgrade, such as a fresh coat of paint or new upholstery?

LOVING GOD

- Visit www.prayingincolor.com and Pray In Color for your prayer list.

A New Creation

Your Whole Life
Body, Soul, and Spirit

W E ARE NOW BEGINNING OUR LAST WEEK IN THIS SESSION. This means that you have had the grace to take a day at a time to complete eleven weeks of doing your very best to eat right, to live well, and to love God.

You have done a great job. By now you look different, you feel different, and you are different—but you may have realized that the journey has just begun. Don't worry: the grace will be there to continue on this road. After all my dieting years, I

> B y now you look different, you feel different, and you are different— but you may have realized that the journey has just begun.

have a better understanding of this process to wholeness. The word *diet* must be taken from my brain, and the phrase *eating right* must take its place. The process feels very familiar, the results are as positive in every way, but the understanding I have is different.

The last week of spiritual readings will talk about loving God and what that really means. Remember the reason we called this book *Your Whole Life?* "Your faith will make you whole" was the promise we saw in God's Word. May God give you the gift of faith to do what you have to do, say what you have to say, let go of what you have to let go of, and hold on fast to what you need.

Maintenance:
The Forgotten Side of Change

I f you have achieved some of your desired goals for balancing your whole life, congratulations! We hope that you have made good progress toward better health in spirit and in mind as well as in body. **The most important thing you can take away from the 3D plan is a decision that your whole life is indeed just beginning, and that you will not go back to old habits and old ways of thinking.**

Be aware that the maintenance of new habits is an important phase of the change process, and that it also requires vigilance and grace. If you know what is necessary and keep pressing on, then it's likely that you will continue to eat a healthy diet, you will create discipline in your lifestyle, and you will enter into discipleship with a loving God. To help you do this, I urge you to remain committed to your support group or to a community of people you trust.

Maggie Davis

For testimonials from others, go to
www.3DYourWholeLife.com
Add your own comments and stories, as well!

Week 12 Daily Devotionals

Theme for the Week DISCIPLESHIP

Verse to Memorize *If any man would come after me,
let him deny himself and take up
his cross daily and follow me.*
—LUKE 9:23

Day 1 What Must I Do?

READ | Mark 10:1–31

And Jesus looking upon him loved him, and said to him, "You lack one thing; go, sell what you have, and give to the poor, and you will have treasure in heaven; and come, follow me." (v. 21)

Of course, *everything* we have been discussing over these weeks is about discipleship—that is, about taking up our own crosses and following after our Lord Jesus Christ. So, it seems appropriate that, through this final week of reflections, we give this idea some focus of its own.

"What must I *do?*" this wealthy young man asks Jesus. How ordinary the question . . . and how extraordinary the answer! We are not surprised that Jesus tells the man to "come, follow me." The unexpected thing was what Jesus told him to do first: "go, sell all that you own, and give it to the poor." First, go . . . then come. The ultimate goal set before this man was to be a disciple—a student, a follower—of Jesus Christ. The "discipline" required of him— to give away that which was so dear to him—was a means to that end. It was not itself the end!

No discipline is meant to be an end in itself. The sacrifice that

Jesus asked of this man was specific to his particular condition. It was, so to speak, his personal price of admission, but it was not the sole purpose of his life. The going and doing were but introductory steps to the coming and following. In other words, disciplines do not make us disciples. *Jesus* makes disciples, and he uses disciplines to assist us on the way.

It turns out that Jesus' wealthy inquirer really had two things with which he did not want to part. For one, he certainly did not want to give away all he owned. At that request, he turned away sorrowful. However, it appears that he possessed an "invisible treasure" that may have been of even more value to him. And, by his words, he displayed that treasure before Jesus. From my youth, he said, I have kept all the commandments— in other words, I have acted the *right* way, I have been a *good* person; there cannot possibly be anything more I need to do. But Jesus saw right through him and lovingly said, no, there is one more thing you need to do; by doing it, you will humbly admit that you do not have all the answers, and that you have much, much more to learn. The "one more thing" that Jesus asked of the man represented his giving up his entirely self-sufficient way of life, and that was the real deal breaker.

What must you and I do to follow Jesus Christ? In principle, the answer is the same for all of us, but it will take a very personal and specific form for each of us. Jesus knows the location of every treasure room in our hearts, and, in order to make disciples of us, he will eventually ask us to empty any that do not hold him as their most valuable possession.

REFLECT | *"You lack one thing," Jesus said to the man. What "one thing" is God asking you to put aside so that you can freely follow him? Or, put another way—what is Jesus asking you to "go and do" so that you can better "come and follow"?*

Day 2 Counting the Cost

READ | Luke 14:15–35

Whoever does not bear his own cross and come after me, cannot be my disciple. For which of you, desiring to build a tower, does not first sit down and count the cost, whether he has enough to complete it? (vv. 27–28)

How many projects have you started with good and fervent intention, only to find that, after a few days or weeks, when the work grew wearisome and the initial vision grew clouded, you "put down your tools" and walked away? How many resolutions have you made, only

to break them within days of their beginning? With determination, the heart says, "I know what I'll do." In discouragement, the body says, "Enough of that." The price of success grows heavier than we first estimated, and so we put aside the load altogether.

Counting the cost: what can that mean? Many of those who set out upon their spiritual lives with a "gung-ho—I can do this" attitude find themselves lagging within a few months. It is little wonder that people regard the fresh enthusiasm of a new Christian with some skepticism ("let's see if *this* lasts"). In his classic devotional book *The Imitation of Christ*, Thomas à Kempis wrote, "We should renew our purpose daily, and should stir up ourselves to fresh enthusiasm, as though this were the first day of our conversion, and we should say, 'Help me, Lord Jesus, that I may persevere in my good purpose and in Your holy service to my life's end. Grant that I may now, this very day, perfectly begin, for what I have done in time past is as nothing.'"[6]

Jesus did not quibble over the "price" of being his Father's Servant. He knew full well what his faithfulness would cost him. Even held within the constraints of human flesh, he counted that cost and, with generous heart and open hand, he paid the full price.

"Though he was in the form of God, [he] did not count equality with God a thing to be grasped, but emptied himself" (Philippians 2:6–7). There is no easy, cheap way to Christian discipleship, and our Lord himself is the prime witness to that truth. He leads the way, by taking up his cross and laying down his own life for our sakes. In turn, he cautions all who would come after him that there is a fixed cost for finishing their course. They, too, must live . . . and die . . . as he did.

Of course, God helps us in our weaknesses; his grace is sufficient for our need, and he provides us with every blessing. We are not required to come up with the cost of discipleship on our own. God is like the father who places a coin in the hand of his son or daughter, so that the child can go and buy a Father's Day gift! What we *are* required to do, however, is to hand over *all* those coins. Every day Jesus asks us to start again, to carry through, to go all the way. No turning back! That's the key.

REFLECT | *In order for you to be his disciple today, what particular price is Jesus asking of you? From time to time, what price just seems too steep for you to pay?*

Day 3   Let Us Hold True

READ | Philippians 3

Only let us hold true to what we have attained. (v. 16)

Given the distance he has come, the amount he has done for the sake of the Kingdom, and the time he has been a faithful disciple, Paul admits to his readers that, still, he has not yet arrived at the goal. "Not that I have already attained this or am already perfect," he says to the Christians in Philippi. This is all the more reason, he tells them, to "strain forward" and to "press on." And one key to such determination, he concludes, is to "hold true" to all that has thus far been attained.

The Philippian church is not in big trouble. There seem to be no major upheavals, no scandals, and no great heresies threatening to destroy the faith of these disciples. What they seem to be in need of, however, is the encouragement not to let go of what they have achieved thus far, together with the assurance that God will not let go of them. "I am sure," affirms Paul, "that he who began a good work in you will bring it to completion at the day of Jesus Christ" (1:6). With serene confidence in the strength of that promise, he can then instruct them to "press on toward the goal."

Through the discipline and obedience of these recent weeks, what have *you* attained? Through your Christian life to this point, what things do you know to be true? What must you hold fast and never give up, in order to "press toward the goal"? The answers to those questions are the stepping-stones for the next leg of your journey. Not wanting to lose what we have gained thus far can be a worthy and powerful motive for moving forward. Wherever we are on our course of discipleship, whatever plateau we may have reached in our upward climb, we need to remember how easy it is to grow lax, to let ourselves go, and to allow old habit patterns of thought and feeling to dominate us once again.

Much change has already taken place in our lives, just as it had in the lives of the Philippians. But, we are not naïve enough to believe that we have obtained final victory. The same temptations, which lured us onto wrong paths in the past, still lie in wait for us today. The same weak points of our human nature are vulnerable to attack, and our thoughts and feelings can still be carried away in hurtful patterns of self-love or self-hate. Familiar battles remain ours to fight, against feelings of jealousy, the desire to control others, judgmental thoughts, and nursed resentments.

For the sake of attaining the final prize in the end, we must hold on today to what we have attained thus far. And how do we do that? We recall and give thanks for what God has done in our lives; we accept the reality of our weaknesses and count on the reality of God's strength; we steadfastly keep our eyes on Jesus and allow him free reign to shepherd us through every situation of our lives; we remain obedient to the light we have been given and open to more light that is yet to come; we do not give up in the face of adversity; and we do not despair when we fail. These are some of the things to which we hold fast . . . and never let go.

REFLECT | *What have been the benefits of daily discipline in your life? How can you keep from letting old habit patterns of thoughts and feelings dominate you again?*

Day 4 Take My Yoke Upon You

READ | Matthew 11

Come to me, all who labor and are heavy-laden, and I will give you rest. Take my yoke upon you, and learn from me; for I am gentle and lowly in heart, and you will find rest for your souls. For my yoke is easy, and my burden is light. (vv. 28–30)

As we think about the *cost* of discipleship, we need also to remember the *promise* of discipleship. Discipleship, says Dietrich Bonhoeffer, means joy. "The command of Jesus is hard, unutterably hard, to those who try to resist it. But for those who willingly submit, the yoke is easy, and the burden is light. *His commandments are not grievous* (1 John 5:3). The commandment of Jesus is not a sort of spiritual shock treatment. Jesus asks nothing of us without giving us the strength to perform it.

His commandment never seeks to destroy life, but to foster, strengthen, and heal it."[7]

Taking the next steps to follow Jesus Christ always means coming under the yoke of his authority in our lives. The ox is yoked for labor so that it can easily be directed by its master's hand. Our yoke is our submission to Jesus, to be guided in all things by him. As we know, he himself was subject to his Father in all things. When Jesus says, "Take *my* yoke upon you," he is completely familiar with the burden he is asking us to bear. He is requiring nothing more (or less) than what was required of him during his days of earthly service. Jesus found his joy and satisfaction in being directed by the Father. The more completely we subject ourselves to him, the more complete will be the rest we find for our souls.

This seems contradictory to reason, doesn't it? "I can be happier by doing someone else's will rather than by doing my own? I can be more peaceful with someone else's yoke around my neck and someone else's burden upon my back rather than my own?" The answer, of course, is a resounding *yes*, but only when that "someone else" is Jesus Christ. "Our hearts are restless," prayed the great fourth-century church teacher Augustine, "until they find their rest in thee." The fruitless searching of his rebellious youth ended when he finally gave his life to God. After looking to everything else to satisfy the longing of his heart, he found that the only rest, true rest, was to be found in subjection to the Lord Jesus Christ.

Jesus Christ is the fulfillment, but discipleship is the path to that deep and abiding "rest" for which all our souls long. We make our way along that path, our wills being conformed more and more to his will, until, one day, we attain true lowliness of heart—when our wills and Jesus' will are one and the same.

REFLECT | *Name those places in your life where you are uneasy, where you long for peace and rest. What connection do they have to also wanting your own way about something? What are you discovering as you submit yourself to Jesus more and more?*

Day 5 Discipleship—Daily

READ | Luke 9:7–27

And he said to all, "If any man would come after me, let him deny himself and take up his cross daily and follow me." (v. 23)

What is discipleship? Learning to will what God wills; learning through pain and failure, through victory and joy, that the ways of heaven are better than our own; dying daily to the demands of the old nature, allowing one's self to be crossed out in exchange for the life of the Spirit (as John the Baptist said of Jesus, "He must increase, but I must decrease" [John 3:30]); giving up the selfish demand that things go the way one wants them to go—all this is discipleship.

What is discipleship? Setting one's hand to the plow and never turning back; pressing forward to a deeper understanding and acceptance of God's truth; further repenting for what we do and why we do it; depending more absolutely upon the grace of God while striving more fervently to work out one's salvation (Philippians 2:12)—all this is discipleship.

What is discipleship? Renewing daily one's love for and loyalty to the One who died that we might live; following where he leads us and going and coming as he directs us; trusting in his steadfast love and rejoicing in his never-ending patience; holding onto one another all the way to the end—all this is discipleship.

Luke is among those who record Jesus' succinct call to discipleship: "take up your cross daily and follow me." Many are the days when we do not want to take up that cross, or *any* cross, for that matter. We have had enough of the struggle. We are tired of fighting against that "old Adam" (or Eve) within us. Frankly, we would rather give in to all the old feelings and give way to all the old choices! How much simpler it would be. . . . But would it? Really?

Beware, disciple! Remember that Jesus said "daily." Taking up our crosses can be compared to the Israelites' gathering their manna—it has to be done freshly every day (Exodus 16:14–21). Yesterday's faithful choices can *assist* us with today's, but they cannot *be* today's. The list above, of all the things that discipleship means, is an inventory for every day, and especially for those days when we would rather put off their burden until tomorrow, or the next day, or the next. *Now* is the day of salvation, said Paul (2 Corinthians 6:2). *Today*, let us take up our cross.

REFLECT | *When are you most tempted to lay aside the weight of your cross? What part(s) of your daily cross would you most like to put down and not have to take up again?*

Day 6   Do As I Have Done

READ | John 13:1–35
For I have given you an example, that you also should do as I have done to you. (v. 15)

Notice what Jesus did in preparation for washing the feet of his disciples. John tells us that he "rose from supper, laid aside his garments, and girded himself with a towel" (v. 4). Through all of these actions, culminating in his bending down to wash and wipe the feet of each of his friends, Jesus took on the role of a servant. He did what any slave at that time would do at the direction of his master. While the host reclined at table, the servant washed the dusty, weary feet of the guests as they prepared to take their meal. But, wait. Isn't Jesus the host of this supper? Didn't he offer the invitations and give all the directions for where and how the meal was to be prepared? How is it that the Host is dressed in a towel? Why is he the one who stoops down and kneels before each of his guests? Isn't this the Lord of all heaven and earth who is holding and washing the feet of these sinful men?

From the beginning to the end of Gospels, we have this strange paradox pictured before us—the lowliness of the Most High, the servanthood of the Master, the self-emptying of the I Am. In his birth, in his life, and in his death there is manifest in Jesus this strange mixture of lowliness and glory. What does this mystery have to do with our discipleship? When he finished his humble task, Jesus said to his disciples, "I have given you an example, that you also should do as I have done to you." At least two conclusions may be drawn from this.

First, we look to the life of Jesus, not only for our salvation, but also for the pattern for our own lives. He is our Lord as well as our Savior. He has lived as we are called to live. Writing to encourage a scattered and persecuted young church, the writer of the First Letter of Peter says: "For to this you have been called, because Christ also suffered for you, leaving you an example, that you should follow in his steps" (2:21). Following in the steps of Jesus, which will surely mean suffering at times, is central to what it means to be a disciple. This may be self-evident, but it is still important that we remind ourselves: if we want to know what it means to live for God, we look at the life of Jesus.

Second, Jesus gave his disciples (and, therefore, us) a very particular example on that eventful night in the upper room. By setting aside his own rank and rights (who *should* have been serving whom?), Jesus loved his disciples. He preferred what was best for them to what was most comfortable for himself. He set aside his rightful office of Teacher and Lord in favor of being their servant. He did something that none of his followers was yet humble enough to do. In all this, Jesus loved them, and, in doing so, he gave them the perfect example of how they were to love one another.

REFLECT | *These days, in what particular way do you need most to be like Jesus? When you consider Jesus' example of love, whose feet do you need to "wash"? What do you need to "lay aside" in order to do so?*

Day 7   A Fruit-bearing Branch

READ | John 15:1–11

By this my Father is glorified, that you bear much fruit, and so prove to be my disciples. (v. 8)

Amidst all of the instructions about obedience, the exhortations to persevere, and the admonitions against being unfaithful, it might be possible to forget that the way of discipleship is, first and foremost, about a *relationship*. All the methods and teachings and disciplines we can possibly follow are really of no value whatsoever unless, first, like branches attached to the vine, our lives are attached to Jesus Christ. That relationship is the only credible beginning and the only worthy end of the disciple's life.

Yesterday, we discussed the example of love that Jesus gave his disciples as they were gathered in the upper room, before they ate supper together. Today's reading is taken from the teaching he gave them after they had finished the meal. The dreadful hours that followed immediately upon these words would eventually lead to Jesus' betrayal, and suffering, and death. His message about bearing fruit, therefore, takes on a special significance in light of these impending events.

Jesus uses the imagery of a grapevine and all its fruit-bearing branches to describe the nature of the relationship he enjoys with his disciples. Like branches attached to their trunk, the disciples' lives are vitally connected with the life of their Lord. He is the source of everything that nourishes and strengthens them. Their only hope of existence, in fact, is found in unbroken attachment to him.

As a branch that abides in the vine, therefore, there are two things that a disciple can most surely expect: to bear fruit, and to be pruned. In fact, says Jesus, both of these things are convincing *proof* that one is a disciple of Jesus Christ. And both of these things are what the past twelve weeks have been about. The victories you have tasted, and that others have tasted with you, are fruits of your discipleship, fresh evidence that your life is attached to Jesus Christ. The pain that you have endured, and that others have endured with you, are signs of skillful pruning, certain confirmation that the Vinedresser is at work in your life.

Discipleship: the pruning of branches and the bearing of fruit. By this God is glorified, and our joy is made full.

REFLECT | *What are some of the fruits of discipleship that you have tasted in recent weeks? Where has some of the pruning been taking place? What do you do from here?*

The Next Step of the Journey

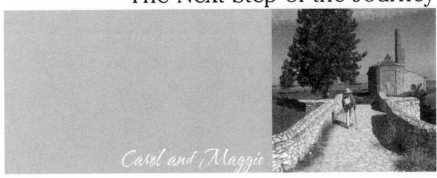

Carol and Maggie

AT THE BEGINNING OF THIS BOOK, I mentioned that I had recently been on a pilgrimage and had found it to be a beautiful experience of eating right, living well, and loving God. Now, at the end of these twelve weeks, I would like to tell you a little more of what I experienced on that trip.

I was alone for seven out of the twenty-one days. There were two towns I wanted to visit that were not on the schedule of the larger group, and so I decided to spend a week on my own. It was a big decision for me, though an extrovert, to travel in Europe by myself— but in my heart, I knew it was God's will, and I felt peaceful about the decision.

You have been on a similar journey over these last twelve weeks. You have confidence that God led you to *Your Whole Life—The 3D Plan.* You are perhaps excited, peaceful, and scared all at the

> You are perhaps excited, peaceful, and scared all at the same time.

same time—just as I was on my pilgrimage. You have found some hard places and have had to make some difficult choices, and they haven't always been comfortable. In fact, I'm sure there were times you simply felt very alone. Sometimes you may have questioned why you got into this "food" thing again.

I experienced those same emotions during my week alone. I got on the wrong train twice. I didn't speak the language, and very few people on the train spoke English. Those were frightening moments, but I discovered that the God who led me was still with me and could even point me in the right direction on the wrong train! I had conversations with God, and I knew I heard his voice over my fears: "I am with you. Do not be afraid." I knew those familiar Scripture verses, and they really came alive when I took the wrong train! I found myself asking God where I should go each moment of the day. Questions that I would have asked members of my travel group, the tour leader, or my husband, I was forced to ask of God, leaning on God alone.

I experienced conversational prayer in a new and deeper way. As I sat on a terrace in a lovely hotel in Umbria, Italy, alone, watching one of the most beautiful sunsets I had ever experienced, I found myself asking God, "What is this all about, Lord?" And I felt his words say in my heart, "It's about you and me, Carol." I felt peace and a sense of gratitude that I have rarely experienced. A smile crept across my face, and a tear rolled down my cheek. "It's all about you and me, Lord." How wonderful! What a privilege to walk and talk and be with God and know beyond a shadow of doubt that God has the answer to every need I have, and he wants more than anything for me to live a whole and holy life!

YOU HAVE COME TO THE END OF THE FIRST TWELVE WEEKS OF THIS NEW PLAN FOR EATING RIGHT, LIVING WELL, AND LOVING GOD. It has, no doubt, been a mixture of joy and pain, success and failure, fun and work. But in it all, you have been walking with God.

I encourage you to see this as a beginning and not an ending. Take out your journal and sit for a half-hour or an hour, and write the things that have meant the most to you. Write the new things you have learned about yourself, and the memory verses that you now know by heart (without looking back). Write a list of the things you have learned about eating right. Don't be worried about what you can't remember. Just write down the practical helps you know will become part of your life now.

What are you going to do in the area of living well? Will you keep counting steps? Will you join a book club, paint a room in your house, take more walks and enjoy the scenery, or connect with family and friends by letters or phone calls? Write those thoughts down, as well.

And how can you practice loving God more? Make him part of every thought and every conversation. My grandmother used to have a plaque that read, "Christ is the unseen guest at every meal, the silent listener to every conversation." May we believe that, and live it.

YOU ALSO NEED TO MAKE A FEW MORE TANGIBLE DECISIONS. There are more materials available for you to continue in the 3D plan. We would love to see you continue with your group, or start a new one. Come visit our website, e-mail us, or call our offices (1-800-451-5006). Keep going in this new direction, and let us support your journey. It would be a joy and a privilege to continue walking with you. There is so much more to learn.

John 12:26 says, *"If any one serves me, he must follow me; and where I am, there shall my servant be also; if any one serves me, the Father will honor him."* This is both a warning and a promise.

First, these words of Jesus are a warning. If we are to serve Jesus, we must follow him. It is not a matter of being good, doing the right thing, obeying the Law, or doing good works. It is a matter of following the living Christ. He is alive, he has a will for us, and he is present with us. Let this reality become more and more a part of your daily consciousness. And when you fail (and we all do), know that he is always there and is always ready with forgiveness and mercy. So pick yourself up, and begin again!

Let us follow the example of Brother Lawrence, a cook in a French monastery in the seventeenth century. He learned a wonderful secret, since retold many times in the little book *The Practice of the Presence of God.* He says,

I occupy myself solely with keeping myself in God's holy presence. I do this simply by keeping my attention on God and by being generally and lovingly aware of Him. This could be called practicing the presence of God moment by moment, or to put it better, a silent, secret and nearly unbroken conversation of the soul with God. . . .[8]

Second, these words of Jesus are a promise. Jesus says, "If any one serves me, the Father will honor him." That is his promise, and you can depend on it. Everyone who truly serves and loves the Son is honored by the Father himself. What greater reward could we ask? What greater invitation could there be to the way of God's love.

As we end, this is my prayer with you and for you:

Thank you, Father, for the challenges and the joys
of these past weeks. Thank you for beginning
a new work of grace and love in my life.
Bless me and those who have journeyed with me,
and grant us grace to go on,
knowing that the way leads home.

In Jesus' Name.
Amen.

Acknowledgments

MANY THANKS to Martin Shannon for revising the daily devotionals that appear in this book. The words that have flowed from Fr. Martin's pen have given inspiration for my whole life.

Initial and Quarterly Health Assessment

date	WEEK 1	WEEK 13
Height/Weight		
Body Mass Index*		
Waist Circumference**		
Hip Circumference**		
Waist to Hip Ratio**		
Clothing Sizes		
Body Fat Percentage (if available)		
Blood Pressure		
Blood Sugar		
Total Cholesterol		
HDL Cholesterol		
LDL Cholesterol		
Triglyceride		
Medications You Take		
Other Health Concerns/ Risk Factors		
Your Purpose & Motivation Now		
Your Short Range Health Goals		
Your Whole Life Goals		

* See BMI Chart on page 275
** See Waist & Hip measurements instructions on www.3DYourWholeLife.com

WEEK 26	WEEK 39	WEEK 52

Body Mass Index (BMI) Chart

The Body Mass Index (BMI) is a way of using your height and weight to identify your risk and to track your progress as you make changes.

To use the following table for U.S. standard measurements, find the appropriate height in the left-hand column labeled Height. Move across to a given weight (in pounds). The number at the top of the column is the BMI at that height and weight. Pounds have been rounded off.

BMI Categories:
- Normal weight = 18.5–24.9
- Overweight = 25–29.9
- Obesity = BMI of 30 or greater

A convenient calculator for both U.S. standard and metric measurements can be found at http://www.nhlbisupport.com/bmi/bminojs.htm.

(Thanks to the National Heart Lung and Blood Institute for the table shown here.)

BODY MASS INDEX TABLE

	Normal						Overweight					Obese										Extreme Obesity														
BMI	19	20	21	22	23	24	25	26	27	28	29	30	31	32	33	34	35	36	37	38	39	40	41	42	43	44	45	46	47	48	49	50	51	52	53	54
Height (inches)																	**Body Weight (pounds)**																			
58	91	96	100	105	110	115	119	124	129	134	138	143	148	153	158	162	167	172	177	181	186	191	196	201	205	210	215	220	224	229	234	239	244	248	253	258
59	94	99	104	109	114	119	124	128	133	138	143	148	153	158	163	168	173	178	183	188	193	198	203	208	212	217	222	227	232	237	242	247	252	257	262	267
60	97	102	107	112	118	123	128	133	138	143	148	153	158	163	168	174	179	184	189	194	199	204	209	215	220	225	230	235	240	245	250	255	261	266	271	276
61	100	106	111	116	122	127	132	137	143	148	153	158	164	169	174	180	185	190	195	201	206	211	217	222	227	232	238	243	248	254	259	264	269	275	280	285
62	104	109	115	120	126	131	136	142	147	153	158	164	169	175	180	186	191	196	202	207	213	218	224	229	235	240	246	251	256	262	267	273	278	284	289	295
63	107	113	118	124	130	135	141	146	152	158	163	169	175	180	186	191	197	203	208	214	220	225	231	237	242	248	254	259	265	270	278	282	287	293	299	304
64	110	116	122	128	134	140	145	151	157	163	169	174	180	186	192	197	204	209	215	221	227	232	238	244	250	256	262	267	273	279	285	291	296	302	308	314
65	114	120	126	132	138	144	150	156	162	168	174	180	186	192	198	204	210	216	222	228	234	240	246	252	258	264	270	276	282	288	294	300	306	312	318	324
66	118	124	130	136	142	148	155	161	167	173	179	186	192	198	204	210	216	223	229	235	241	247	253	260	266	272	278	284	291	297	303	309	315	322	328	334
67	121	127	134	140	146	153	159	166	172	178	185	191	198	204	211	217	223	230	236	242	249	255	261	268	274	280	287	293	299	306	312	319	325	331	338	344
68	125	131	138	144	151	158	164	171	177	184	190	197	203	210	216	223	230	236	243	249	256	262	269	276	282	289	295	302	308	315	322	328	335	341	348	354
69	128	135	142	149	155	162	169	176	182	189	196	203	209	216	223	230	236	243	250	257	263	270	277	284	291	297	304	311	318	324	331	338	345	351	358	365
70	132	139	146	153	160	167	174	181	188	195	202	209	216	222	229	236	243	250	257	264	271	278	285	292	299	306	313	320	327	334	341	348	355	362	369	376
71	136	143	150	157	165	172	179	186	193	200	208	215	222	229	236	243	250	257	265	272	279	286	293	301	308	315	322	329	338	343	351	358	365	372	379	386
72	140	147	154	162	169	177	184	191	199	206	213	221	228	235	242	250	258	265	272	279	287	294	302	309	316	324	331	338	346	353	361	368	375	383	390	397
73	144	151	159	166	174	182	189	197	204	212	219	227	235	242	250	257	265	272	280	288	295	302	310	318	325	333	340	348	355	363	371	378	386	393	401	408
74	148	155	163	171	179	186	194	202	210	218	225	233	241	249	256	264	272	280	287	295	303	311	319	326	334	342	350	358	365	373	381	389	396	404	412	420
75	152	160	168	176	184	192	200	208	216	224	232	240	248	256	264	272	279	287	295	303	311	319	327	335	343	351	359	367	375	383	391	399	407	415	423	431
76	156	164	172	180	189	197	205	213	221	230	238	246	254	263	271	279	287	295	304	312	320	328	336	344	353	361	369	377	385	394	402	410	418	426	435	443

Source: Adapted from *Clinical Guidelines on the Identification, Evaluation, and Treatment of Overweight and Obesity in Adults: The Evidence Report*

Recommended Daily Portion Guidelines

food group	calories/serving	800	1000	1200	1400
Vegetables (cups)	25-50	2	2	3	3
Fruits (cups)	80	1	1	1	1.5
Whole Grains (1 oz)	80	2	3	3	3
Starches (1 oz)	80	0	0	0	1
High Calcium Foods (1 oz or 1 cup)	100	1.5	1.5	2	2
High Protein Foods (1 oz or 1 cup)	60-100	3	3	4	4
Oils & Other Fats	50	1	2	3	4
Water (8 oz)	0	5	5	6	6

		800	1000	1200	1400
Core Food Calories		705	835	1035	1205
Your Choice Calories		100	150	175	175
Total Calories		805	985	1210	1380

1600	1800	2000	2200	2400	2600	2800	3000
3	3	3	4	4	4	5	5
1.5	2	2	2	2	2	2.5	2.5
3	3	3	3	4	5	5	5
1	2	3	4	4	4	4	5
3	3	3	3	3	3	3	3
5	6	6	6	7	7	7	7
5	5	6	7	7	8	9	10
7	7	8	8	9	9	10	10

1420	1605	1735	1900	2045	2175	2295	2425
175	200	250	300	350	400	500	550
1595	1805	1985	2200	2395	2575	2795	2975

Guidelines for Leading a 3D Group

FOLLOW THESE SIMPLE STEPS, and keep in touch with Carol and Maggie by visiting www.3Dyourwholelife.com.

1 INITIATE THE FORMATION OF YOUR GROUP by asking people to focus on the next 12 weeks. The 3D program is designed for making and measuring progress in 12-week segments. Each group member should commit to coming together once per week for at least that length of time.

2 EVERYONE IN THE GROUP needs to have their own copy of *Your Whole Life*. Carol Showalter and Maggie Davis will walk with you and present thoughts and challenges for your journey. Spiritual readings for every day of the first 12 weeks are also included in the book.

3 SELECT A LEADER OR A TEAM of leaders for your group. If your group is originating in your congregation, the leader or leaders can be appointed by the pastor; in other situations, they should be selected by the members of the group. This position is one of facilitating the group, including ordering materials, finding the best time for the meeting, starting and ending the group, and showing an extra amount of care for each person in the group as needed. In many instances, the first person that reads *Your Whole Life* or somehow discovers the 3D Plan is the person that goes to her pastor and to her friends, works to get a group started, and automatically becomes the leader. This is actually a wonderful way to start a group. It is important to remember that the leader is a part of the group and should be seen as equally involved in the journey.

4 EACH 3D GROUP should be no larger than 12 people.

5 Try to keep your weekly meeting time to a one-hour session. The time should be divided into three sections:

> ■ **The first 20 minutes**—Prayer. Then discuss the eating section of the book and allow time for each member to speak about progress, struggles, and new challenges.

> ■ **The next 20 minutes**—Discuss how you have lived well this week.

> ■ **The final 20 minutes**—Discuss how you loved God this week, look ahead to the goals of the week to come, ask questions of each other, and share answers. One of the most important tools of a successful 3D group is the art of listening; refrain from trying to fix every problem that comes up. Pray.

6 Finally, every group member who has joined the program to lose weight should be encouraged to weigh in weekly, and to share their results and be supported by the group.

R EMEMBER THAT THERE ARE NO FAILURES in a 3D group. Do your best to understand this in a new and encouraging way. If a person learns only one Scripture verse every week for 12 weeks, she now loves God more successfully. If another person has begun to take a walk every other day, she is successfully learning about living well. And if others have learned more about eating right, whether or not they have had much weight loss thus far, they too are successful. Success in 3D is NOT measured in pounds.

New materials are available to continue the journey.
Visit www.3DYourWholeLife.com
—a resource for you throughout the 12 weeks.

Notes

1. Readers outside the United States may not use Calories as measurements of energy. Several tools for converting from calories to joules, the metric unit of energy, are available online. Many of the charts in this book are available at www.3DYourWholeLife.com with measurements shown in Calories and kilojoules.
2. Jamieson, Fausett, and Brown, *Commentary Critical and Explanatory on the Whole Bible*. Originally published in 1871, this commentary can be found on several websites, including the Christian Classics Ethereal Library at http://www.ccel.org/ccel/jamieson/jfb.html.
3. J.B. Phillips, *The New Testament in Modern English* (London: G. Bles, 1958).
4. Earl Jabay, *The Kingdom of Self* (Plainfield, NJ: Logos International, 1974), 27.
5. David Brown, *Critical, Experimental and Practical Commentary*, vol. 6 (Grand Rapids, MI: Eerdmans, 1945), 264.
6. Thomas à Kempis, *The Imitation of Christ*, ed. Hal M. Helms (Brewster, MA: Paraclete Press, 1982), 30.
7. Dietrich Bonhoeffer, *The Cost of Discipleship*, rev. ed. (New York: Macmillan, 1963), 40.
8. Brother Lawrence, *The Practice of the Presence of God*, trans. Robert J. Edmonson (Brewster, MA: Paraclete Press, 1985), 93.

The 3D Prayer

Dear Lord,
This is a new day
That means I can expect from your hand
    all I need to live.
Help me to know
Your grace is sufficient
Your power is overwhelming
    and your peace and joy are here for the asking.
I need you in so many practical ways, Lord
I need you to help me choose the right spirit
    at the beginning of the day
I need you to help me with my family
    the work I need to get done
    and the pressures that come at me
    before my eyes are even open.
I need you to go ahead of me every step of the way
You will do that
This day is yours
I am yours.
Thank you for loving me and giving me
    the gift of life today.
When I am ready to close my eyes
    at the end of this day
May I say with a steady voice:
I have loved you more today than I did yesterday
But not as much as I will tomorrow.
Make it so, dear Lord.
Amen.